DIAGNOSTIC MANUAL OF
TUMOURS OF THE CENTRAL NERVOUS SYSTEM

To Fiona

Experience is the name every one gives to their mistakes
Oscar Wilde

When you have excluded the impossible whatever remains, however improbable, must be the truth
Sir Arthur Conan Doyle

To let a hundred flowers bloom and a hundred schools of thought contend is the policy for promoting the progress of the arts and sciences
Mao Tse-Tung

DIAGNOSTIC MANUAL OF TUMOURS OF THE CENTRAL NERVOUS SYSTEM

Antony J. Franks

BSc MB ChB MRCPath

Honorary Consultant Neuropathologist, General Infirmary,
Leeds; Lecturer in Pathology, University of Leeds;
Former District Medical Officer (Outer Islands),
Republic of Kiribati, Central Pacific

CHURCHILL LIVINGSTONE
EDINBURGH LONDON MELBOURNE AND NEW YORK 1988

CHURCHILL LIVINGSTONE
Medical Division of Longman Group UK Limited

Distributed in the United States of America by
Churchill Livingstone Inc., 1560 Broadway, New York,
N.Y. 10036, and by associated companies, branches
and representatives throughout the world.

First published 1988

ISBN 0-443-03524-5

British Library Cataloguing in Publication Data
Franks, Antony J.
    Diagnostic manual of tumours of the central nervous system.
    1. Central nervous system – Tumours – Diagnosis
    I. Title
    616.99′28075   RC363

Library of Congress Cataloging in Publication Data
Franks, Antony J.
    Diagnostic manual of tumours of the central nervous system.

    Bibliography: p.
    Includes index.
    1. Central nervous system – Tumors – Diagnosis –
Atlases. 2. Histology, Pathological – Atlases. I. Title.
[DNLM: 1. Central Nervous System Diseases – diagnosis.
2. Nervous System Neoplasms – diagnosis. WL 358 F834d]
RC280.N43F73 1988   616.99′28   87-11658

Produced by Longman Group (FE) Ltd
Printed in Hong Kong

PREFACE

Standard texts of pathology of central nervous system tumours of necessity provide an account of their characteristic features. Whilst the range of appearances (sometimes extraordinary) that can occur within a single tumour or between tumours of the same type may be emphasised, the diagnostic implications of this variability are often such that the non-specialist who turns to the text for assistance may come away with less rather than more confidence. The increasing demand for rapid diagnosis by cryostat sections and smears in neurosurgical practice means that often the young pathologist is faced with unfamiliar material in an unfamiliar medium presenting unfamiliar appearances, unlike textbook illustrations of paraffin sections which, in routine practice, are not usually available for at least 18 hours.

This book is designed to provide a practical 'bench manual' for use by trainees (in both neuropathology and general pathology) and experienced pathologists who only occasionally have to deal with neuropathological material. It aims to demonstrate the differences (and similarities) that are seen when the same tumour type (and in many cases the same specimen) is examined in smears, cryostat sections and paraffin sections. Correlations are made between these various appearances and intrinsic tumour structure, and those features that are of value in arriving at a diagnosis are emphasised.

Consideration is given to common and less common neoplasms, as well as some lesions (frequently cystic) which, although not neoplastic, frequently present as tumours in neurosurgical practice. All the material illustrated is derived from diagnostic biopsies and is representative of the kind of preparations on which diagnoses will be made.

Selected references are given which should provide either a review of the lesion under consideration or serve as the basis for more detailed reading. The selection is to some extent a personal one, with more references being given for those tumours which are of intrinsic interest or the centre of current controversy. Space is also provided for the recording of personally examined cases that may be of interest for teaching or research purposes.

Although primarily intended for pathologists I hope that this book will be of interest to neurosurgeons and radiotherapists, both experienced and in training, and that the contents may stimulate further research into more effective diagnosis and management of this biologically diverse and technically challenging group of lesions.

Ilkley, 1988   A.J.F.

ACKNOWLEDGEMENTS

Many people have contributed to the compilation of this book, both wittingly and unwittingly, but always willingly and it is a pleasure to acknowledge their assistance.

I am indebted to Dr Denis Harriman for suggesting this project and for his encouragement during its uncertain initial stages. For the loan of material for photography I thank Dr Alex Gordon and Dr Jeanne Bell in Edinburgh (Figs. 9.1–9.3), Dr David Piercy in Hull (Figs. 2.80, 4.1 and 4.14) and Dr James Ironside in Leeds (Figs. 7.6 & 13.1). Philip Bogue, Elizabeth Wakefield, Caroline Plummer, David Blythe and Christine Iddon in the Neuropathology Laboratory of the University Department of Pathology provided unfailing (and uncomplaining) technical assistance, and Pete Walsh and Christine Atkin provided help with the electron microscopy. Ah-Lien Guest and Des Tyrrel spent hours organising records and finding cases and Steve Toms mounted endless transparencies and produced black and white prints. Dr Mike Dixon and Dr James Ironside provided helpful criticism and proof reading assistance, and Dr Ciaran O'Brien advised on the current classification of lymphomas. My sincere thanks to them all. I also wish to thank all those trainees in pathology who, on attachment to the Neuropathology Department, asked the questions which this book now attempts to answer. I hope it does so more adequately than I did at the time.

The staff of Churchill Livingstone gave invaluable assistance and tolerantly accommodated my wishes.

I owe an especial debt of gratitude to Dr James MacKenzie, to whom the contents of this book will be only too familiar, for much fruitful and stimulating discussion working out diagnostic principles, and for his invaluable comments on the final product.

Finally I thank my wife Fiona, and my children Simon and Katharine, who have put up with my absence and my presence during the production of this book, who helped and, above all else, understood.

Ilkley, 1988   A.J.F.

TECHNICAL NOTE

This book was written on a BBC model B microcomputer using Wordwise Plus and Interword wordprocessors (Computer Concepts).

All photomicrographs are reproduced from original transparencies taken on Kodak Ektachrome EPY ASA 50 Professional film using a Zeiss Photomicrosope III with a Wratten 82B filter.

In the figure legends the following abbreviations are used:

AB   Alcian Blue
AB/PAS/D   Alcian Blue, Periodic Acid/Schiff after Diastase
CAM 5.2   Antibody against low molecular weight cytokeratins
CP   Cryostat specimen after paraffin processing
CS   Cryostat section
ChS   Churukian Schenk
CYTO   Cytospin preparation
EM   Electron Micrograph
EMA   Epithelial Membrane Antigen
GFAP   Glial Fibrillary Acidic Protein
GIEM   Giemsa
HGH   Human Growth Hormone
HE   Haematoxylin and Eosin
IP   Immunoperoxidase indirect immunostaining
OG   Orange G
ORO   Oil Red O for neutral lipid
PAS   Periodic Acid/Schiff
PS   Paraffin section
RETIC   Gordon and Sweet's method for Reticulin
S-100   S-100 protein
SP   Smear preparation
TP   Touch preparation

Sources of commercial antisera:

EMA, GFAP, HGH, Kappa Light chains and S-100: Dakopatts. Dako Ltd, 22 The Arcade, The Octagon, High Wycombe, Buckinghamshire, HP11 2HT

Cytokeratins (CAM 5.2): Becton-Dickinson Laboratory. Impex Ltd, Lion Road, Twickenham, Middlesex, TW1 4JF

CONTENTS

1 TECHNIQUES OF RAPID DIAGNOSIS

2 SMEAR PREPARATION

Two main techniques are available for the rapid diagnosis of biopsies from central nervous system tumours. These are the cryostat section and the smear (and its variant—the touch, or dab, preparation). Decisions as to which technique to use are usually determined by the nature of the tissue submitted and specimen size. If the specimen is very small a smear is more likely to yield useful information, whereas a tough tumour may only yield cells for study if firmly 'dabbed' on to a slide with a pair of forceps. Whenever the specimen is large enough cryostat sections should also be prepared, if possible from the same tissue fragment from which the smear specimens were taken.

The relative values of the smear and cryostat techniques for diagnostic purposes will vary with experience and the tumour under consideration. For the trainee in general pathology or neuropathology, and for those who only occasionally handle neurosurgical material both should be used in a complementary fashion since each provides unique information. Whilst the expert may rely on one or the other it is sensible to gain experience of both in the context of the same lesion, thus making interpretation easier and learning more efficient.

With the growing use of fine needle aspiration for diagnosis in fields other than neurosurgery the skills acquired in examining and interpreting smear preparations in the light of simultaneous cryostat sections will aid the transition from one medium of investigation to the other.

Most pathologists are so used to interpreting Haematoxylin and Eosin (HE) stained sections that in this book their routine use for both smear and cryostat sections is advocated. The extra time involved is more than justified by the increased ease of interpretation. Other stains that might be used to aid diagnosis on smears or cryostat sections are Toluidine Blue to demonstrate mucin, or lipid stains such as Oil Red O. Extra sections or smears can also be prepared for subsequent immunohistochemical or immunocytochemical studies, or tissue can be fixed for electron microscopy if the case appears to warrant it.

Smears

The results of smearing a tissue fragment will reflect the varying proportions of vascular or stromal elements to parenchymal tissue, and the degree and nature of cell-to-cell adhesion. Cells with little or no cohesion (eg lymphomas) will spread easily into single cells, whereas those with strong attachments via intervening external lamina (eg neurilemomas) will spread little, if at all, to yield tissue fragments (Fig. 1.3) with few if any separated cells. Tissues whose component cells form widespread but relatively weak cell attachments (eg carcinomas or meningiomas) will result in a mixture of cell sheets, smaller cell clusters or separated individual cells. Where the cell contacts are via processes (eg astrocytomas or ependymomas) these will be drawn out in the smearing process so that they are clearly visible in the thinned smear and their presence will also be apparent on any individual cells separated from the larger masses.

Whilst a smear may accentuate a papillary architecture (eg choroid plexus papilloma) any tumour with a prominent vasculature (which resists smearing) and easily spread neoplastic cells will tend to demonstrate a papillary vascular orientation. Even so the appearances taken in conjunction with cytological detail may be suffiently characteristic to be of diagnostic value (eg ependymoma).

Examination of the edges of tissue fragments will allow a ready assessment of the degree of separation of single cells or small cell groups, and in these areas cell detail is best seen. If a tumour does not smear well and if single cells are not separable then the cytological information obtainable will be limited, but the way it smears will, in itself, be a valuable piece of information and aid diagnosis.

Whenever possible samples to be smeared should be taken from the same piece of tissue that is used for cryostat sections. Where multiple specimens are submitted wider sampling can more easily be achieved with smears from several pieces than with cryostat sections. A tumour fragment (roughly 1 mm³) is placed at one end of a glass slide and then divided into smaller pieces (Fig. 1.1), each of which is transferred to a new slide. This method is far easier than attempting to remove pieces ready to smear directly from the biopsy specimen.

The single specimens are lightly squashed by a second slide held at right angles but with surfaces parallel and this second slide is then drawn along the length of the first slide (Fig. 1.2), the two surfaces still being held parallel. The smear is then fixed in 95% ethanol and stained (Fig. 1.3). (Rinse in water; Gill's No.3 Haematoxylin 2 mins; rinse; differentiate and blue in weak ammonia-water; rinse, counterstain 1% Eosin 30 secs, wash; dehydrate; mount).

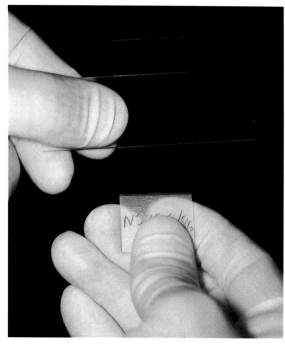

Fig. 1.2 The degree of compression necessary will vary with the tissue and is best learned by experience. In this case the left hand is making the smear.

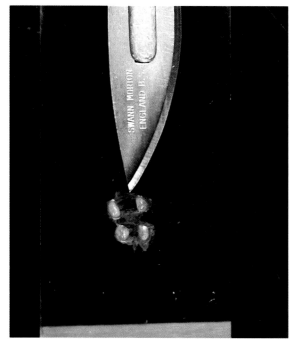

Fig. 1.1 The approximate size of a tissue fragment to be smeared can be judged by comparison with the scalpel blade and the slide width.

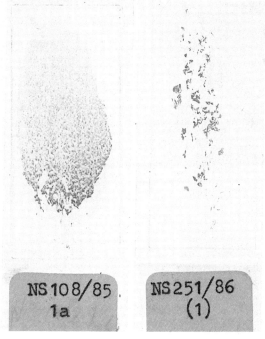

Fig. 1.3 A uniformly spread smear from a malignant glioma (left) contrasts with a fragmented smear from a neurilemoma (right).

4 CRYOSTAT SECTIONS

Cryostat sections have a rather 'woolly' appearance due to the absence of the fixation effect that is in part responsible for the 'crisp' cell boundaries and fine nuclear detail seen in routine paraffin sections. The lack of the shrinkage effect of paraffin processing makes cells look larger and exaggerates anisocytosis. Whilst these facts may be of little concern when dealing with epithelial or lymphoid tissues, in the context of CNS tumour diagnosis they may make essential structures hard to see and emphasise minor tissue components (eg stromal cells in haemangioblastoma). Despite these disadvantages the cryostat section provides information about the architecture of the tissue and serves as a bridge between the cytological detail of the smear and the mental picture of the tumour based on paraffin sections.

The major artefact to be aware of in the preparation of cryostat sections is ice-crystal formation (Fig. 1.4) that results when slow freezing allows ice-crystals to form within the tissue and distort its structure. Factors that predispose to this are inefficient freezing, specimens that are too large, and the immersion of tissue in saline in the operating theatre. Ideally the specimen should be no more than 3 mm in thickness and a maximum of 1 cm diameter, although the latter dimension will be determined by the size of the microtome chuck. Many neurosurgical biopsies will be within this size range and will not require further manipulation.

The practice of sending specimens immersed in saline should be discouraged. It is sufficient to place the specimen on a piece of gauze that has been first wetted with saline and then wrung out so it is merely damp. If the gauze is then folded over the specimen and enclosed in a screw top bottle or Petri dish it will survive transport over considerable distances without problems.

It cannot be stressed too highly that where a diagnosis depends on the findings of material examined in one medium, the findings in the other medium, even if not diagnostic, must be compatible. Thus, for example, a misdiagnosis of astrocytoma on a cryostat section of a piece of neurilemoma (p. 80) will be avoided. This also applies to the misinterpretation of technical artefact without reference to other findings (Figs. 1.4–1.6).

Close co-operation with the surgeon providing the biopsy is essential, and it often helps to determine the exact purpose for which the rapid examination is being carried out. Where further intra-operative management depends absolutely on the nature of the tumour, as accurate a diagnosis as possible should be provided and material requested as necessary to achieve this end. Lesser levels of certainty are required intra-operatively where the information may determine postoperative management, especially if there is subsequent clinical deterioration. In these cases confirmation of a neoplastic process may be required, or information as to whether a tumour is benign or malignant, intrinsic or extrinsic, but not necessarily its exact histological type. On occasion the surgeon may simply require confirmation that a burrhole biopsy has removed abnormal tissue that will be adequate for diagnostic purposes when submitted to full paraffin processing, thus avoiding the need for the further biopsy that would follow a negative result.

It follows from this that it is necessary to be familiar with normal tissues likely to be encountered in the course of a neurosurgical procedure. This familiarity can be gained by study of archive material, or by the preparation of smears from normal brain tissue obtained at autopsy. This will prevent errors such as mistaking normal neuronal satellite cells for infiltrating tumour cells (Fig. 2.8), cerebellar granular layer for medulloblastoma (Fig. 4.3) or choroid plexus for papillary carcinoma (Fig. 14.8).

Clinical information concerning the age and sex of the patient and site of the lesion must always be available. Provision of a diagnosis in isolation may be misleading for the surgeon, embarrassing for the pathologist and dangerous for the patient.

Artefact

Extensive ice crystal artefact in the preparation of a cryostat section (Fig. 1.4) has resulted in a loose appearance bearing a strong superficial resemblance to an astrocytoma. The smear however shows cells with an epithelial appearance (Fig. 1.5) quite unlike those expected in an astrocytoma. Preparation of a fresh specimen shows the acinar structure of an adenocarcinoma (Fig. 1.6) which was confirmed on subsequent paraffin sections.

Discrepancies between smear and cryostat sections may result from sampling, but this can be avoided by ensuring that, wherever possible, both preparations are made from the same tissue fragment. Cryostat sections are much more prone to artefacts that may result in misdiagnosis and in such circumstances more weight should be placed on the smear appearances. If doubt remains and there is sufficient tissue it is better to repeat the cryostat section taking all precautions to avoid artefact.

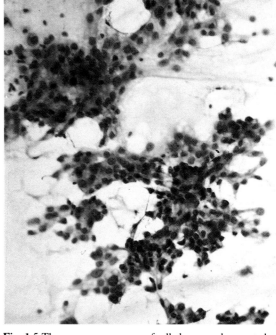

Fig. 1.5 The smear appearances of cell clumps and separated cells with malignant features are totally incompatible with the diagnosis of astrocytoma. × 205

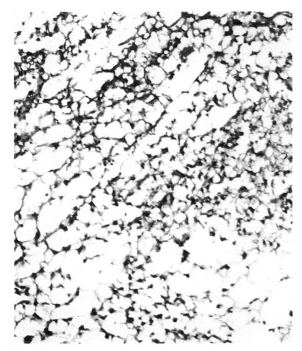

Fig. 1.4 Architectural disruption by ice-crystal artefact resembles an astrocytoma but should be recognised at an early stage and such sections discarded. × 128

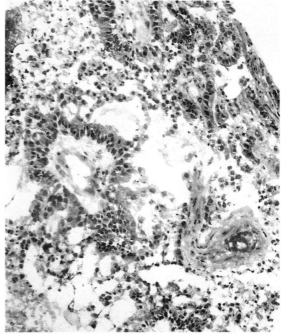

Fig. 1.6 A repeat cryostat section free of artefact shows a totally different appearance that is now compatible with the smear picture. × 128

The basic classification of central nervous system tumours follows standard practice and is based on its normal elements. The major subdivisions are tumours of glial, meningeal, nerve sheath and lymphoreticular origin, with separate consideration being given to tumours of primitive neuroectodermal cells, neurones, germ cells, pineal parenchymal cells, blood vessels and paraganglia. Other lesions that do not derive from intrinsic normal elements or that develop from misplaced tissues include craniopharyngiomas and metastatic tumours. There have been a number of different attempts to provide an agreed classification of brain tumours that have received their impetus from the need to provide information that accurately conveyed the nature and (more importantly) the likely behaviour of a lesion. Whilst these classifications usually agree on the major divisions, there has frequently been disagreement over the definition of tumour subtypes. This problem is compounded by the heterogeneity of astroglial tumours and the frequency with which a tumour contains areas of two supposedly separate subtypes.

It is important to realise that although the histology of a tumour may give an indication of its histogenesis and its likely behaviour, other factors such as tumour site and resectability, patient age and available therapy may have a far greater bearing on outcome. This book does not aim to provide a definitive classification, but instead utilises one that has been found in practice to provide surgical colleagues with information of value. It most closely follows that of the Armed Forces Institute of Pathology fascicle on Central Nervous System Tumours (Rubinstein 1972).

The commercial availability of antibodies that allow the demonstration of specific antigens in paraffin sections by the immunoperoxidase method has provided a valuable tool for the diagnosis of central nervous system tumours. Such antibodies are of most value when histologically similar tumours are known to have clear differences in antigen expression but sometimes combinations of antigen expression will have to be assessed. Due to variations in specificity of antibodies from differing sources it is wise to stain control tumours under local conditions before accepting published reactivities or using new antibodies for diagnostic purposes.

FURTHER READING

Adams JH, Graham DI, Doyle D 1981 Brain biopsy. The smear technique for neurosurgical biopsies. Chapman and Hall, London

Burger PC, Vogel FS 1982 Surgical pathology of the nervous system and its coverings, 2nd edn. John Wiley, New York

Escourolle R, Poirier J 1978 Manual of Basic Neuropathology, 2nd edn. Saunders, Philadelphia

Lantos PL 1983 Histochemistry of the tumours of the nervous system. In: Filipe MI, Lake BD (eds) Histochemistry in Pathology, Churchill Livingstone, Edinburgh, ch. 8, p. 70–81

Moss TH 1986 Tumours of the nervous system. An ultrastructural atlas. Springer Verlag, London

Rubinstein LJ 1972 Tumors of the Central Nervous System. Atlas of Tumour Pathology, second series. Fascicle 6. Armed Forces Institute of Pathology, Bethesda, Maryland

Rubinstein LJ 1982 Tumors of the Central Nervous System. Atlas of Tumour Pathology, second series. Supplement to Fascicle 6. Armed Forces Institute of Pathology, Bethesda, Maryland

Russell DS, Rubinstein LJ 1977 Pathology of Tumours of the Nervous System, 4th edn. Edward Arnold, London

Weller RO 1984 Colour Atlas of Neuropathology. Oxford University Press, Oxford

Zulch KJ 1979 International histological classification of tumors No. 21. Histological typing of tumours of the central nervous system. World Health Organisation, Geneva

2 GLIAL TUMOURS

The pattern of infiltration seen in astrocytomas (benign or malignant), glioblastoma multiforme and oligodendroglioma is frequently sufficiently characteristic for a diagnosis of infiltration by a glioma to be made even though primary tumour structure is not represented in the biopsy specimen. This is especially important in exploratory operations where the material for initial study frequently derives from the edge of the tumour rather than its centre, and an early distinction between intrinsic and metastatic tumour is of value to the surgeon. Although a similar type of infiltration does occur in ependymomas (p. 43) it is usually less obvious and rarely of particular value in diagnosis.

The boundary between gliomas and adjacent brain is ill-defined due to the diffuse infiltration of single cells into the neuropil in contrast to the clear margins that exist between metastatic tumours and adjacent brain. This results in a diffuse increase in cellularity that can be appreciated on both sections and smears (Figs. 2.1 & 2.2) and emphasises the need to be familiar with the normal cellularity of brain tissue (Fig. 2.3) although this does vary from area to area. Prominence of glial elements, especially astrocytes, will also occur in reactive states and must be distinguished from neoplastic infiltration. A real or apparent increase in astrocytes may be due to an increase in size of cells, or an increase in their number, or both. Reactive enlargement of astrocytes is seen in the context of white matter oedema (from whatever cause) without increase in numbers, whereas increase in astrocyte numbers (true gliosis) may be associated with reaction to infection, ischaemia or nonglial tumours (Fig. 2.4). The glial response to ischaemia is usually more marked if there is associated haemorrhage which may also evoke proliferation of vascular elements and heighten the resemblance to a malignant glial tumour. Astrocytic proliferation in response to ischaemia is usually accompanied by a loss of neurones (which generally survive at the edge of infiltrating gliomas) or by macrophages containing lipid derived from degenerating myelin. These latter are not usually a feature of infiltrating glial tumours unless adjacent brain has been rendered ischaemic by vascular compromise due to local or generalised increases in intracranial pressure.

There are no absolute criteria by which reactive astrocytes can be distinguished from neoplastic cells, although abnormal mitoses or aberrant nuclear morphology (Fig. 2.5) are better indications of a neoplastic nature than cell size. The most useful distinguishing feature is their relationship to pre-existing structures.

A common effect of a rapidly expanding intracranial tumour, whether an intrinsic infiltrating glioma, a metastasis, or an extrinsic lesion such as a meningioma, is oedema of the white matter. This results from changes in vascular permeability and may be responsible for a significant proportion of the space occupying effects of an intracranial tumour, and biopsies from the edge of an infiltrating glioma may therefore consist solely of oedematous white matter.

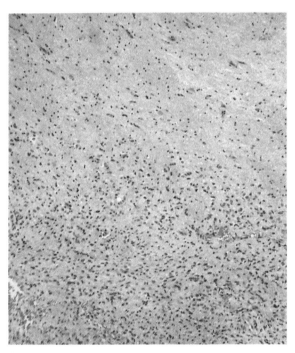

Fig. 2.1 Edge of glioblastoma multiforme. (M 59) Infiltration by glioma results in an ill-defined margin between normal brain (top) and tumour (below). PS HE × 80

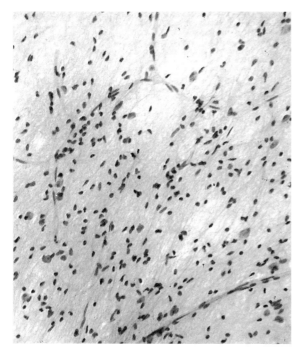

Fig. 2.2 Edge of oligodendroglioma. (F 41) The excess cellularity of the cortex is due to diffusely infiltrating tumour cells. SP HE × 205

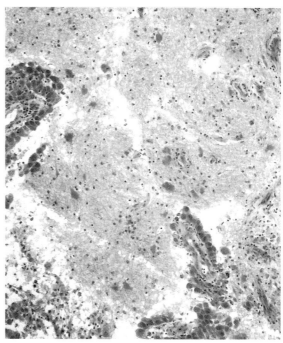

Fig. 2.4 Metastatic carcinoma. (M 64) Reactive astrocytes stain intensely in brain adjacent to, but well demarcated from, tumour. CS HE × 100

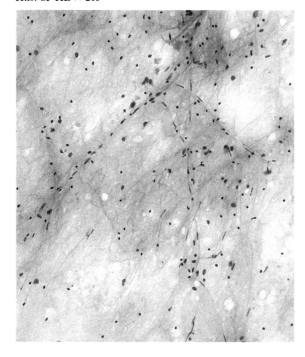

Fig. 2.3 Normal cortex. (M 42) The normal cellularity can be compared with that seen in Fig. 2.2. SP HE × 128

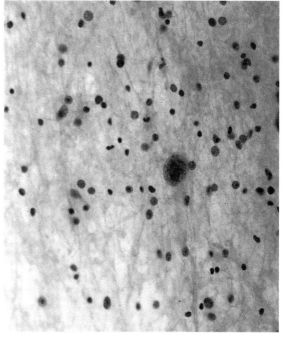

Fig. 2.5 Edge of astrocytoma. (F 30) Large atypical nucleus in white matter without visible cytoplasm is extremely suspicious of tumour. SP HE × 320

It is a characteristic of glial tumours that they infiltrate adjacent brain as single cells following planes within the tissue and accumulating at physical boundaries. Thus neoplastic glial cells infiltrate along blood vessels (Figs. 2.6 & 2.7) and axons, and accumulate around neurones (Figs. 2.8 & 2.9) and beneath the pia. The architecture that is thus imposed on the tumour cells is termed a secondary structure to contrast with a tumour's intrinsic primary structure. In infiltrating gliomas the boundary between the cortex and underlying white matter may be effaced by tumour cells. This is a useful distinguishing feature from reactive states in which the boundary is usually preserved and in which the increase in astrocytes is generally more diffuse.

The clustering of glial cells around neurones (satellitosis) that is a normal feature of some parts of the cerebral cortex may closely resemble neoplastic perineuronal infiltration. However the latter is usually accompanied by an increase in interstitial cellularity and by perivascular infiltration. Preservation of the boundary between cortex and white matter would be strong evidence against isolated satellitosis being due to infiltration by tumour. Infiltrating cells in perineuronal and other locations may not show the same cytological features as those that make up the bulk of the tumour. Shrinkage artefact may separate them from adjacent structures reproducing an appearance that, whilst it is characteristic of the cells that comprise oligodendrogliomas (p. 36), may also be seen in cells that make up the infiltrating margin of a glioblastoma (Fig. 2.10).

These appearances are characteristic of gliomas, reflecting a pattern of invasion which distinguishes them from metastatic tumours (Ch. 14) although a limited degree of perivascular infiltration may be seen at the edge of some anaplastic carcinomas. It will be apparent that a distinction between a low and high grade glioma, or identification of its cell type, can rarely be made with any confidence solely on the basis of the infiltrating cells.

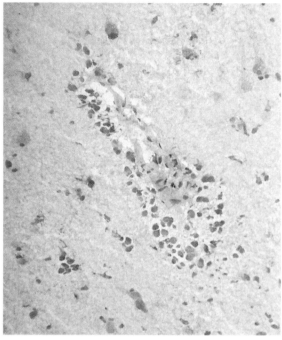

Fig. 2.6 Infiltrating astrocytoma. (M 42) Infiltration of the perivascular space by tumour suggests a glioma even if the type cannot be identified. CS HE × 205

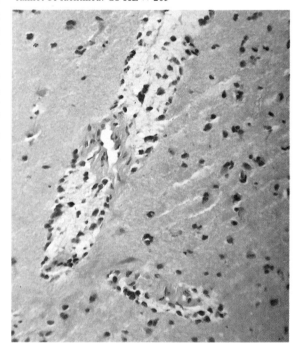

Fig. 2.7 Same tissue as Fig. 2.6. In paraffin sections there is a far clearer contrast between tumour cells and adjacent neuropil. PS HE × 205

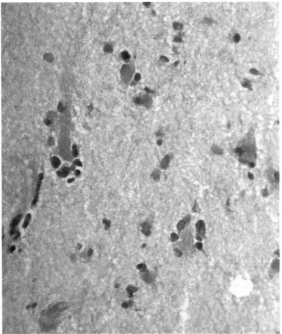

Fig. 2.8 Same case as Fig. 2.6. Mildly pleomorphic cells cluster around neurones in one pattern of glial tumour infiltration. CS HE × 320

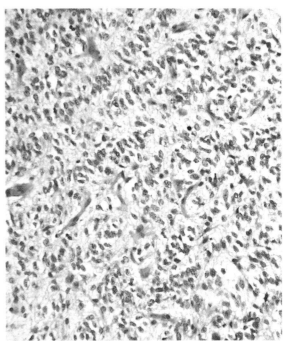

Fig. 2.10 Edge of glioblastoma. (F 47) The alignment of cells, their regular cytology and the tendency to form haloes belies their origin. PS HE × 205

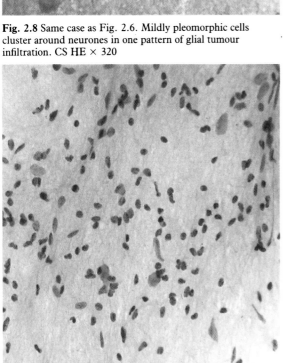

Fig. 2.9 Edge of oligodendroglioma. (M 41) Tumour cells infiltrate the neuropil diffusely but still tend to cluster around neurones (centre). SP HE × 205

Although tumours of astrocytes have certain features in common, they form a heterogeneous group of lesions differing in site, age of occurrence and prognosis. Histological grading systems have been devised to classify tumours in a way that is prognostically useful but there is widespread inconsistency in their application, and the effects of patient age, tumour site and therapy often weigh as heavily in the balance as histology. Nevertheless a division of astrocytic tumours into low and high grade lesions does appear to be clinically useful. Despite their intrinsically infiltrative nature some have a slow enough growth pattern and a cellular histology that sufficiently resembles that of normal astrocytes to be termed benign. These lesions are the low grade astrocytomas with which this section deals. High grade tumours comprise malignant astrocytomas and glioblastoma multiforme which are dealt with separately. In some grading systems the low grade tumours are divided into grades 1 and 2, malignant astrocytoma is designated grade 3 and glioblastoma multiforme grade 4.

Whilst certain histological patterns are commonly found in tumours occurring at a characteristic age or site, the use of a histological term to denote a clinicopathological entity is not useful since the histological appearances are not specific. Some generalisations can however be made regarding the nature and localisation of astrocytic tumours. In adults they are commoner in the cerebral hemispheres and more likely to be solid and histologically uniformly fibrillary or microcystic, while in children they are more likely to be in the cerebellum, to be cystic and to show a mixture of histological patterns. Astrocytomas occur in the brain stem and spinal cord and rare examples of primary meningeal astrocytomas are described arising from astrocytic elements that are sometimes found in normal meninges. One variant, the pleomorphic xanthoastrocytoma shows features that are thought to indicate origin from subpial astrocytes, and another, the astroblastoma, recapitulates the relationship between primitive astrocytes and blood vessels in the developing brain.

The histological appearances of astrocytic tumours reflect the wide variety of forms that non-neoplastic astrocytes can take, although this variety is often less obvious in smear preparations. In general the cytoplasm of astrocytes, even when present in small amounts, is still obvious in cryostat sections with the result that cells can appear to show more anisocytosis than is seen in smears or subsequent paraffin material. Broadly speaking, the appearances of astrocytic tumours depend on the degree and complexity of process formation, the relative proportions of cell body to processes, and the presence and degree of cyst formation. Although one form may pre-

dominate in any individual tumour there is frequently a mixture of appearances and it should be appreciated that the subclassifications used are largely for descriptive convenience. Low grade astrocytomas show little, or only mild, cellular pleomorphism, few if any mitoses, and necrosis and haemorrhage are rare. When seen these features should raise the suspicion of malignant change.

Although tumours in adults may show this histological pattern uniformly, in children it is more commonly encountered as a component of a variegate astrocytic lesion. In a typical fibrillary, or microcystic, astrocytoma the component cells are loosely interconnected by numerous processes with the formation of fine interstitial cysts. The smear shows the relative uniformity of the component cells and emphasises their processes and astrocytic nature (Fig. 2.11). The loose appearance on frozen section is characteristic and the cell processes are not so clearly seen (Fig. 2.12). This latter method of examination tends to emphasise anisocytosis in contrast to the far more accurate representation of cell size provided by a smear and, although necrosis, mitoses and vascular proliferation will be absent, the study of a cryostat section alone may be misleading. In paraffin processed tissue cellular details (especially cell processes) are clearer and the typical microcystic pattern is apparent (Fig. 2.13).

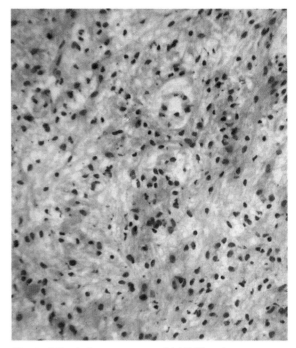

Fig. 2.12 Cerebellar astrocytoma. (M 11) There is more variation in cell density and cell size and the fibrillar background is difficult to see. CS HE × 205

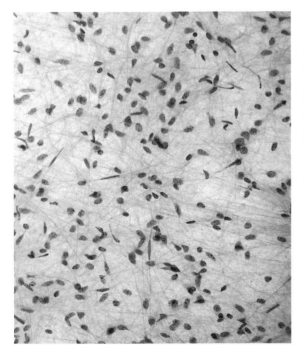

Fig. 2.11 Infundibular astrocytoma. (F 16) Cells of uniform size and spindle shape with fine processes are typical of a low grade astrocytoma. SP HE × 205

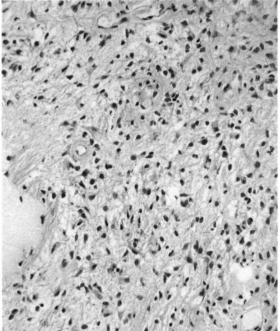

Fig. 2.13 Same case as Fig. 2.12. After paraffin processing the background of tumour cell processes is easier to appreciate. CP HE × 205

In the pilocytic, or piloid, variant (Figs. 2.14–2.20) the cells are more uniformly elongated and have a greater degree of cell-to-cell cohesion with the result that the tissue is less readily smeared (Fig. 2.14). Tumours of this type commonly occur in the infundibular region in children but are not restricted to this site, and in the hemispheres show a particularly indolent behaviour. Frequently the pilocytic areas are interspersed with areas composed of parviprocessed cells (protoplasmic astrocytes) with small regular nuclei and only a small amount of cytoplasm (Figs. 2.15 & 2.16) which on smears may resemble the cells of an ependymoma or oligodendroglioma (Fig. 2.17). Although predominantly solid (Fig. 2.18) such tumours may show cyst formation due to the accumulation of extracellular fluid/matrix between groups of cells. This will be apparent on cryostat (Fig. 2.19) and paraffin sections (Fig. 2.20). A similar appearance may be encountered in subependymomas (p. 45).

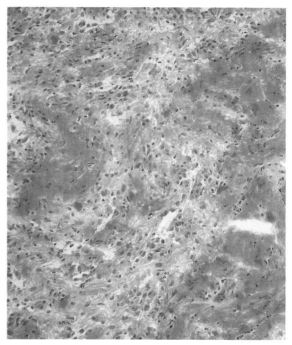

Fig. 2.15 Same case as Fig. 2.14. Dense areas of sparsely cellular tumour with Rosenthal fibres enclose more cellular zones. CS HE × 128

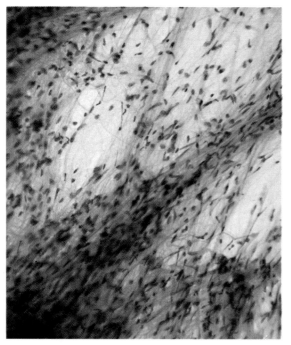

Fig. 2.14 Cerebral astrocytoma. (F 6) Smears are more tenacious and eosinophilic masses of GFAP (Rosenthal fibres) can be seen. SP HE × 205

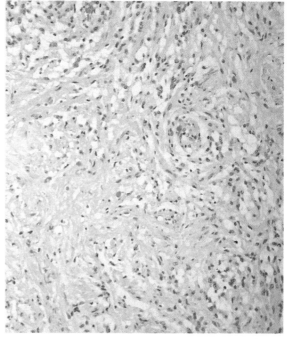

Fig. 2.16 Same case as Fig. 2.14. The contrasts are less obvious after paraffin processing but cellular and sparsely cellular areas are still discernible. PS HE × 128

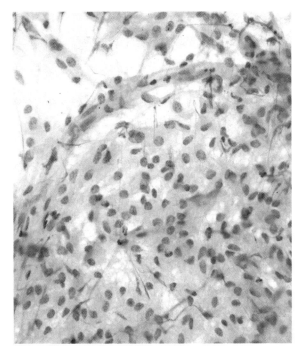

Fig. 2.17 Cerebral astrocytoma. (M 52) 'Protoplasmic' astrocytes show minimal process formation but smear much better than the pilocytic areas. SP HE × 320

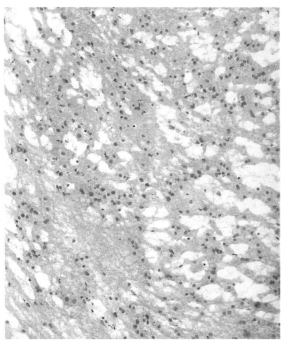

Fig. 2.19 Same case as Fig. 2.17. There is a predominance of fibrillary matrix with cells more widely dispersed than expected from the smear appearances. CS HE × 128

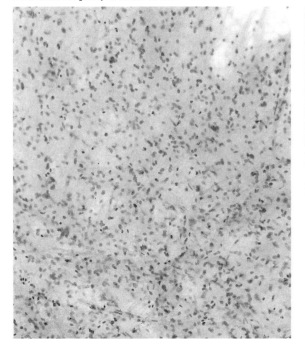

Fig. 2.18 Same case as Fig. 2.17. Tumour cells are coherent, smear poorly and little process formation is visible. SP HE × 128

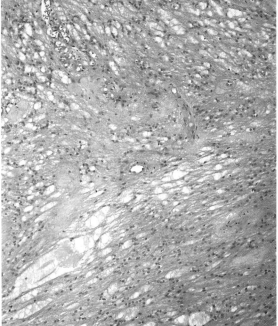

Fig. 2.20 Same case as Fig. 2.17. The basic pattern of intermixed acellular and cellular zones is distorted by the formation of cysts in the former. PS HE × 80

All astrocytic tumours are to some extent variegate in their appearance but this is most apparent in cerebellar tumours in children (Fig. 2.21) and in optic nerve gliomas. The latter frequently show an admixture of fibrillary and pilocytic areas although the contribution made to the appearances by residual non-neoplastic elements is uncertain. This heterogeneity makes it difficult to categorise histological subtypes of astrocytoma in a way that has clinical significance. Although the pilocytic variant in the cerebral hemisphere in adults does appear to be associated with a better prognosis, the location of the tumour and the influence that this has on resectability is probably of as much importance. The available evidence indicates that the use of surgery and radiotherapy in combination offers better prospects for prolonging survival than either treatment used in isolation.

Features that may be seen in astrocytic tumours, irrespective of type, are Rosenthal fibres (Figs. 2.14, 2.30 & 2.31) which are dense aggregates of glial fibrillary acidic protein (GFAP) with an elongated or globular shape, hyaline droplets composed either of GFAP or other cytoplasmic components, and calcium aggregates (Fig. 2.22) which may be sufficiently dense to be apparent on radiographs.

In addition to the microcystic and solid areas described above, blood vessels may be numerous (although not showing the active proliferation that characterises malignant astrocytomas) with areas resembling an angioma (Fig. 2.21). Tumours in which areas of haemangioblastoma (Ch. 7) coexist with astrocytoma are termed angiogliomas but are rare. Cell clusters (resembling perineuronal infiltration) may be a striking, although usually focal, feature (Figs. 2.23 & 2.24). Occasionally such a pattern is intermixed with pilocytic areas (Fig. 2.24) or is found focally in oligodendrogliomas. These clusters of cells (in astrocytomas or oligodendrogliomas) express little or no GFAP (Fig. 2.25) raising the possibility that they are related to the cells that form typical oligodendrogliomas. Mixed tumours of oligodendroglial and astrocytic origin are further considered on page 38.

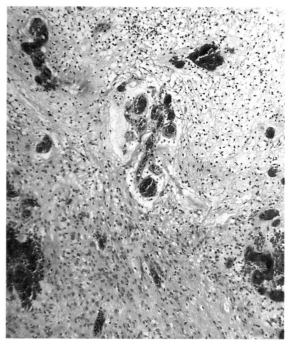

Fig. 2.21 Cerebellar astrocytoma. (M 11) This tumour shows pilocytic areas (below) and microcystic areas (top) and a prominent vasculature. PS HE × 80

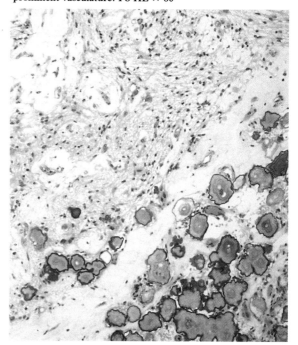

Fig. 2.22 Cerebral astrocyoma. (M 34) Calcium accretions which dominate parts of this field had formed a central mass with surrounding tumour. PS HE × 128

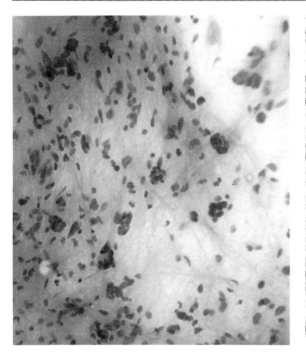

Fig. 2.23 Cerebellar astrocytoma. (M 20) Cell clusters are a conspicuous feature in this lesion and may resemble perineuronal infiltration. SP HE × 205

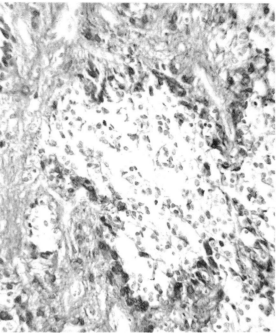

Fig. 2.25 Cerebral astrocytoma. (F 41) GFAP is strongly expressed in the fibrillary areas in marked contrast to the areas of cellular clustering. PS IP × 205

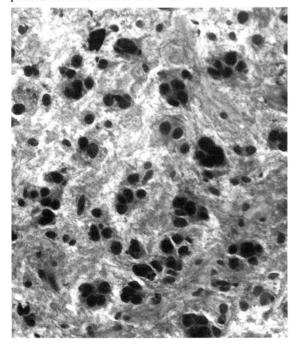

Fig. 2.24 Same case as Fig. 2.23. In sections the clusters can be seen to consist only of tumour cells with sparsely cellular intervening fibrillary matrix. CS HE × 320

The gemistocytic astrocytoma is composed of cells with large amounts of eosinophilic cytoplasm and varying degrees of process formation (Figs. 2.26–2.28). Such lesions are only rarely 'pure' and gemistocytes are often present focally in other astrocytic tumours. Gemistocytic areas may be a focal feature in histologically malignant tumours, and sampling error may underly the observation that gemistocytic astrocytomas frequently behave more aggressively than other astrocytomas. The size and shape of the component cells are often very similar to those of reactive astrocytes and it is with these tumours that small fragments derived from an area of reactive gliosis are most likely to be confused. One feature that may be quite prominent is a lymphocytic infiltrate (Fig. 2.28), although this is by no means exclusive to the gemistocytic astrocytoma.

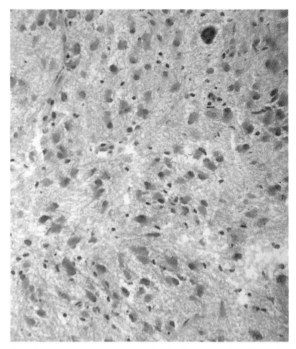

Fig. 2.27 Same case as Fig. 2.26. The intense eosinophilia of cells due to their GFAP content is typical of cryostat preparations. CS HE × 205

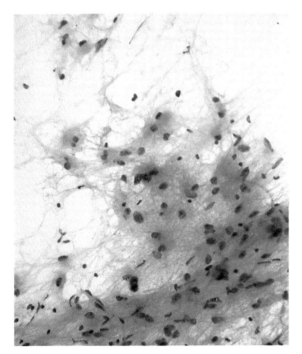

Fig. 2.26 Cerebral gemistocytic astrocytoma. (M 53) Large eosinophilic cell bodies and prominent processes identify gemistocytic astrocytes. SP HE × 205

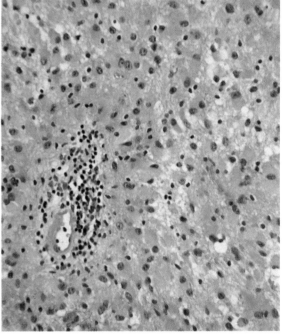

Fig. 2.28 Same case as Fig. 2.26. There is often a prominent interstitial and perivascular population of small lymphocytes in these tumours. PS HE × 205

Although commoner in children these are a histologically heterogeneous group of lesions which have macroscopic cyst formation in common. Coalescence of small cysts in fibrillary (Fig. 2.29) and other astrocytomas may give rise to larger spaces although macroscopic cysts may also develop as the result of fluid leakage from numerous small vessels that can sometimes be found bordering a cyst wall. The large cyst that develops may be responsible for much of the space-occupying effect of the tumour which may be reduced to a peripheral nodule in the cyst wall. Treatment may be confined to drainage of the cyst and biopsy of its wall (Fig. 2.30) which is often just a layer of densely gliotic tissue containing no recognisable tumour. The diagnosis of a neoplastic lesion is presumptive until material from the tumour nodule is available for examination (Fig. 2.31). Such tumour may show a variety of histological appearances, no one being typical of a cystic astrocytoma, although pilocytic and fibrillary patterns are encountered most frequently.

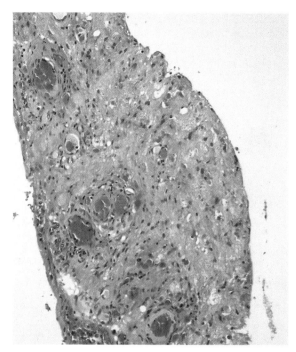

Fig. 2.30 Cystic cerebellar astrocytoma. (M 11) The cyst wall shows intense gliosis and Rosenthal fibres but no identifiable tumour. PS HE × 128

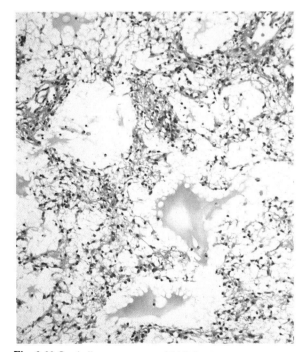

Fig. 2.29 Cerebellar astrocytoma. (F 10) In places the tumour has a microcystic pattern but coalescence has resulted in formation of larger cysts. PS HE × 128

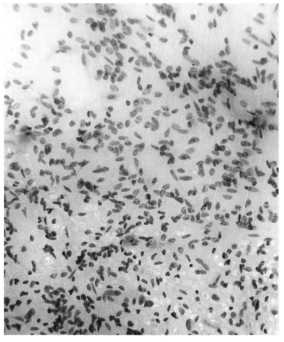

Fig. 2.31 Same case as Fig. 2.30. Tissue from the solid portion of the lesion shows neoplastic astrocytes and numerous Rosenthal fibres. SP HE × 205

This uncommon tumour is usually found in the walls of a cerebral ventricle and is typically (though not invariably) associated with tuberous sclerosis. It is well demarcated from adjacent brain and lacks the insidious infiltration of many astrocytomas. The giant cells that give the lesion its name may raise the possibility of a malignant astrocytic tumour on frozen section (Fig. 2.32) but the appearance of groups of giant astrocytes interspersed with a less cellular fibrillary background and the tenacious smear (Fig. 2.33) that results are not typical of malignant astrocytoma or glioblastoma. Calcification (often apparent radiologically), the paucity of mitoses, and the absence of necrosis and vascular proliferation would also favour a low grade lesion. The resemblance of some of the giant cells to neurones and the presence of neurofilament protein in a few suggests some relationship to the rare ganglioglioma (p. 76). Paraffin sections (Fig. 2.34) show the astrocytic features of the giant cells (such as expression of GFAP) and the absence of the characteristic reticulin pattern (Fig. 4.14) of a ganglioglioma.

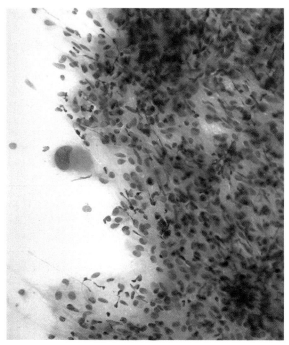

Fig. 2.33 Same case as Fig. 2.32. In smears the presence of a population of smaller cells contrasts with the giant cells. SP HE × 205

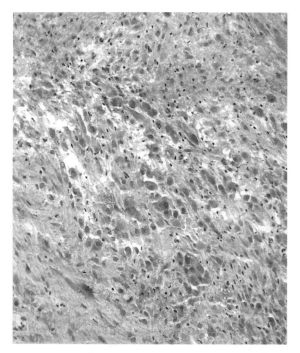

Fig. 2.32 Third ventricle giant cell astrocytoma. (F 30) Large pleomorphic cells dominate the histological picture. CS HE × 128

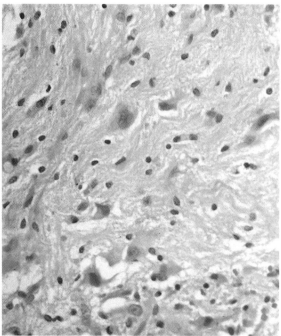

Fig. 2.34 Same case as Fig. 2.32. The giant cells are often clearly astrocytic and lack the Nissl substance seen in neoplastic ganglion cells. PS HE × 320

This is a rare lesion but ignorance of its existence may result in an incorrect diagnosis of malignancy and institution of inappropriate therapy. It has a superficial cortical location, often with quite widespread infiltration of the leptomeninges, and has not yet been described after the fourth decade. The tumour was first identified by virtue of its indolent behaviour despite the extremely worrying cytology. The tumour cells are characterised by their pleomorphic appearance (Figs. 2.35 & 2.36), their lipid content (evidenced by the pale glassy cytoplasm or the demonstration of lipid on frozen sections), and the production of an external lamina by some of them which results in a focal pericellular reticulin pattern (Fig. 2.37). This last feature is shared by the subpial astrocyte from which the tumour is thought to arise. The combination of features described above is diagnostic but it is important to ensure that necrosis and vascular proliferation are absent if the rare glioblastoma in which lipid-containing cells accumulate is not to be confused with a pleomorphic xanthoastrocytoma.

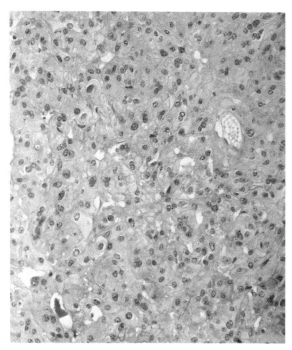

Fig. 2.36 Same case as Fig. 2.35. The 'ground glass' appearance of the cells is a reflection of their lipid content. PS HE × 205

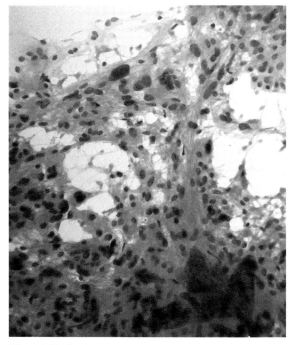

Fig. 2.35 Parietal pleomorphic xanthoastrocytoma. (F 33) The gross cellular atypia and gigantism closely resembles a malignant glial tumour. SP HE × 205

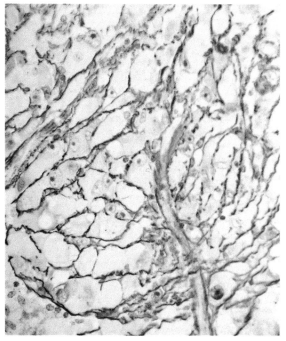

Fig. 2.37 Same case as Fig. 2.35. Pericellular reticulin is typical of this lesion and quite unlike other gliomas. PS RETIC × 320

The diagnosis of this rare tumour is based on a characteristic histological appearance, but controversy surrounds its very existence because similar appearances may be encountered in other glial tumours. It is a lesion of the cerebrum and has been described over a wide age range. The tumour cells are arranged around blood vessels in a pattern that recapitulates the vascular relationships of embryonic astrocytes and is discernible in smears (Fig. 2.38) and cryostat sections (Fig. 2.39). The resulting rosettes (Fig. 2.40) resemble those of an ependymoma but examination of the tumour edges will reveal a typical astroglial pattern of infiltration. A similar perivascular arrangement of cells may be found focally in glioblastomas and gemistocytic astrocytomas, but these will have other typical areas and different smear appearances. Cytologically the cells that are not related to blood vessels show varying degrees of process formation and may resemble the cells of an oligodendroglioma, but unlike the latter they contain GFAP. Calcification may be found in astroblastomas but is not invariable.

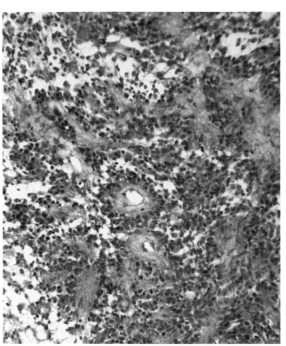

Fig. 2.39 Same case as Fig. 2.38. The resemblance to an ependymoma is obvious and due attention must be given to the smear appearances. CS HE × 205

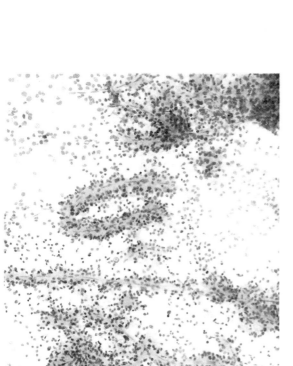

Fig. 2.38 Parietal astroblastoma. (M 6) Cells adhere to vessels but their interstitial separation helps distinguish this tumour from an ependymoma. SP HE × 205

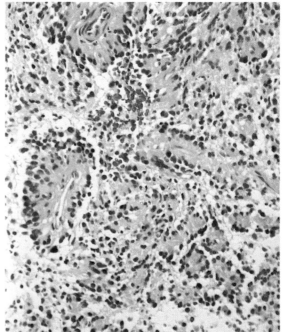

Fig. 2.40 Same case as Fig. 2.38. After paraffin processing the looser arrangement of those cells that are not applied to blood vessels is more apparent. PS HE × 205

FURTHER READING

Albright AL, Price RA, Guthkelch AN 1985 Diencephalic gliomas of children. Cancer 55:2789–2793

Bonnin JM, Pena CE, Rubinstein LJ 1983 Mixed capillary hemangioblastoma and glioma. A redefinition of the 'angioglioma'. Journal of Neuropathology and Experimental Neurology 42:504–516

Bonnin JM, Rubinstein LJ, Papasozomenos S Ch, Marangos PJ 1984 Subependymal giant cell astrocytoma. Significance and possible cytogenetic implications of an immunohistochemical study. Acta Neuropathologica (Berlin) 62:185–193

Clark GB, Henry JM, McKeever PE 1985 Cerebral pilocytic astrocytoma. Cancer 56:1128–1133

Cohadon F, Aouad N, Rogier A, Vital C, Rival J, Dartigues JC 1985 Histologic and non-histologic factors correlated with survival time in supratentorial astrocytic tumours. Journal of Neuro-Oncology 3:105–111

Garcia DM, Fulling KH 1985 Juvenile pilocytic astrocytoma of the cerebrum in adults. A distinctive neoplasm with favorable prognosis. Journal of Neurosurgery 63:382–386

Gheradi R, Baudrimont M, Nguyen JP, Gaston A, Cesaro P, Degos JD, Caron JP, Poirier J 1986 Monstrocellular heavily lipidized malignant glioma. Acta Neuropathologica (Berlin) 69:28–32

Hoag G, Sima AAF, Rozdilsky B 1986 Astroblastoma revisited: a report of three cases. Acta Neuropathologica (Berlin) 70:10–16

Ilgren EB, Stiller CA 1987 Cerebellar astrocytomas: clinical characteristics and prognostic indices. Journal of Neuro-Oncology 4:293–308

Kalyan-Raman UP, Cancilla PA, Case MJ 1983 Solitary, primary malignant astrocytoma of the spinal meninges. Journal of Neuropathology and Experimental Neurology 42:517–52

Kepes JJ, Rubinstein LJ 1979 Pleomorphic xanthoastrocytoma: a distinctive meningocerebral glioma of young subjects with relatively favorable prognosis. Cancer 55:170–173

Taratuto AL, Monges J, Lylik P, Leiguarda R 1984 Superficial cerebral astrocytoma attached to dura. Cancer 54:2505–2512

NOTES

Lesions that are histologically and cytologically clearly astrocytic in nature but in addition show mitoses, cellular pleomorphism and atypical cell forms, should be considered malignant (Figs. 2.41–2.45). These lesions are sometimes referred to as 'anaplastic' astrocytomas but the use of this term in other contexts to indicate complete absence of differentiation results in confusion and the term malignant astrocytoma is to be preferred. Whilst there may be vascular proliferation, the absence of necrosis distinguishes these lesions from glioblastoma multiforme.

Malignant features may be found focally in a tumour with a predominantly low-grade histology, in a recurrent tumour that originally showed a low-grade histology, as a uniform appearance in a newly presenting tumour (Figs. 2.41–2.43) or (most commonly) in a small biopsy from a tumour that on more extensive sampling shows the features of a glioblastoma multiforme. The diagnosis of a malignant astrocytoma should therefore, if possible, be accompanied by an indication as to whether malignant features are focal or uniform. In small biopsies, further sampling may reveal that the appearances are not representative of the tumour as a whole. An astrocytoma showing focal malignant change is likely to have a different prognosis to one with a uniformly malignant histology and there is some evidence that not only do these latter tumours differ in their behaviour from glioblastomas, but that mitotic count and degree of vascular proliferation also correlate with shorter survival times.

In view of the variable appearances of astrocytomas it is not surprising that malignant change, when it occurs, is often focal (Figs. 2.44 & 2.45). In excised low grade tumours a careful search should be made of paraffin sections especially if there was any degree of anisocytosis in smear preparations. This is particularly important in recurrent lesions which have a propensity to gradual transition from a low grade to a high grade tumour.

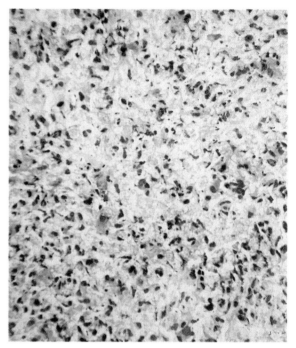

Fig. 2.41 Malignant cerebral astrocytoma. (M 27) Focally high cell density and pleomorphism should prompt a search for other features of malignancy. CS HE × 205

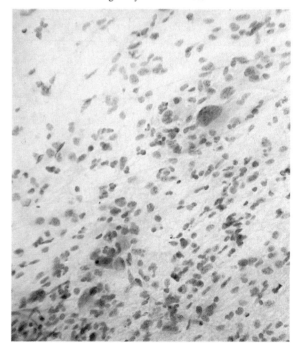

Fig. 2.42 Same case as Fig. 2.41. Atypical cells are seen against a background of pleomorphic cells showing little process formation. SP HE × 205

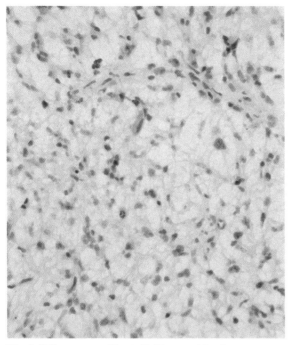

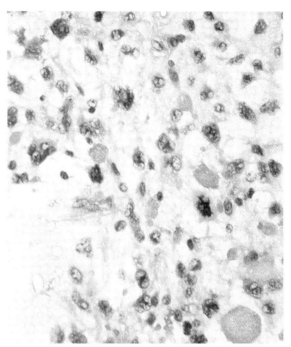

Fig. 2.43 Same case as Fig. 2.41. Pleomorphism is accompanied by mitotic activity, but the lack of necrosis precludes a diagnosis of glioblastoma. CP HE × 256

Fig. 2.45 Same case as Fig. 2.44. Within the cellular area the degree of pleomorphism and the presence of mitoses suggest focal malignant change. PS HE × 320

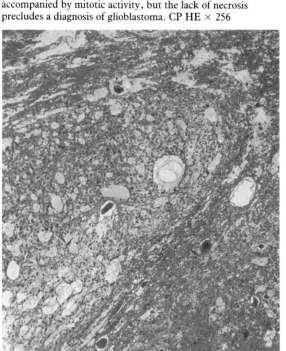

Fig. 2.44 Cerebral astrocytoma. (F 17) An area of higher cell density compresses surrounding, predominantly pilocytic, tumour. PS HE × 32

FURTHER READING

Burger PC 1986 Malignant astrocytic neoplasms: classification, pathologic anatomy and response to treatment. Seminars in Oncology 13:16–26

Cohadon F, Aouad N, Rougier A, Vital C, Rival J, Dartigues JC 1985 Histologic and non-histologic factors correlated with survival time in supratentorial astrocytic tumours. Journal of Neuro-Oncology 3:105–111

Fulling KH, Garcia DM 1985 Anaplastic astrocytoma of the adult cerebrum. Prognostic value of histologic features. Cancer 55:928–931

Nelson DF, Nelson JS, Davis DR, Chang CH, Griffin TW, Pajak TJ 1985 Survival and prognosis of patients with astrocytoma with atypical or anaplastic features. Journal of Neuro-Oncology 3:99–103

NOTES

The glioblastoma multiforme is the commonest glial tumour in adults, and encompasses a wide range of histological appearances which have in common a glial nature, cytological features of malignancy, focal necrosis and proliferation of new vessels (within the tumour and in adjacent brain). As the second part of its name implies the range of cytological appearances is enormous, possibly indicating that a variety of histogenetic origins may underlie these tumours. In practical clinical terms they behave as a relatively homogeneous group although tumours with a predominance of giant cells may be associated with a slightly longer survival. They are frequently cystic due to central necrosis but selection of intact tissue fragments from the semi-fluid contents may provide small pieces of tumour that are quite adequate for diagnosis. The astrocytic lineage of many glioblastomas is evident in smears and cryostat sections (Figs. 2.46 & 2.47) where the process forming nature of the component cells is well demonstrated. Other cytological markers of malignancy are present in the form of cellular pleomorphism and mitoses (Fig. 2.48).

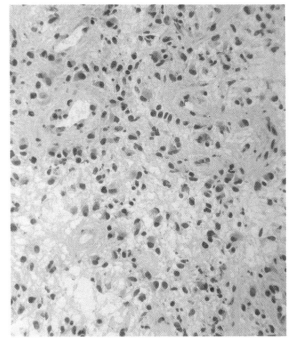

Fig. 2.47 Same case as Fig. 2.46. Pleomorphism, tendency of cells to cluster around vessels and the presence of necrosis are typical findings. CS HE × 205

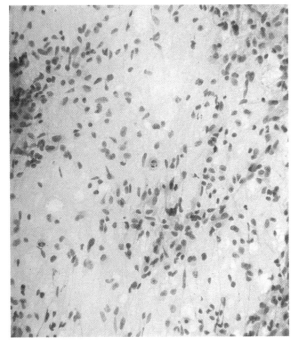

Fig. 2.46 Temporal glioblastoma. (M 54) The cells are recognisably astrocytic although the degree of process formation varies considerably. SP HE × 205

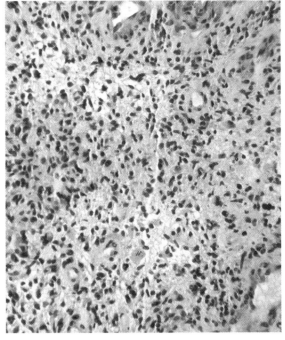

Fig. 2.48 Same tissue as Fig. 2.46. Tumour cells often show a considerable range of sizes and shapes and aberrant mitoses may be common. CP HE × 205

These tumours excite a vigorous proliferative response on the part of vascular endothelium with the result that hyperplastic endothelial buds (Figs. 2.49 & 2.50) and congeries of proliferating vessels (Fig. 2.51) are common. Their main importance lies in the clues they may give to the nature of the tumour, and in the possibility of misinterpreting the proliferating endothelial cells as cells of a metastatic epithelial tumour, especially if mitoses are present. Whilst proliferating vascular tissue may give rise to epithelial-like knots in a smear, the single cells and cell sheets of an epithelial tumour will be absent. Although characteristic of glioblastoma multiforme, vascular proliferation may be found in many rapidly growing lesions, both primary and metastatic, and also in response to haemorrhage.

The abnormal vasculature that develops in a glioblastoma and the inconstant and irregular blood flow through it predisposes to haemorrhage, thrombosis and necrosis. A cardinal feature of glioblastoma, this necrosis often demonstrates a concentration of cells in the border zone between viable and necrotic tumour resulting in a pseudopalisaded appearance (Figs. 2.52 & 2.53). Necrotic tumour may be evident in cryostat sections or smears as granular or amorphous eosinophilic debris sometimes with cell ghosts. When the specimen consists entirely of necrotic material it may be confused with cerebral infarction, but the typical foam cells of the latter are absent (see discussion on p. 8). Very rare examples of granular cell glioblastomas are described but in these there are usually areas with typical histological features. Care should be exercised however when dealing with a biopsy from the edge of a large tumour where shifts may have led to a direct vascular compromise resulting in infarction of brain adjacent to tumour. Here the diagnosis of cerebral infarction rather than tumour does not necessarily exclude the latter and clarification of the site of the biopsy and reassurance concerning its representative nature should be sought.

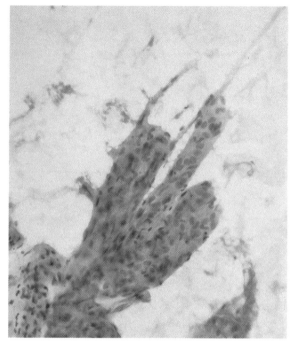

Fig. 2.49 Temporal glioblastoma. (F 62) Proliferation of endothelium may be apparent as solid masses of cells or haphazard sprouts from larger vessels. SP HE × 205

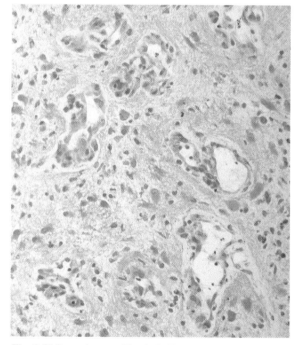

Fig. 2.50 Same tissue as Fig. 2.49. Endothelial hyperplasia and vascular irregularity may be found in tissue adjacent to the tumour as well as in it. CS HE × 205

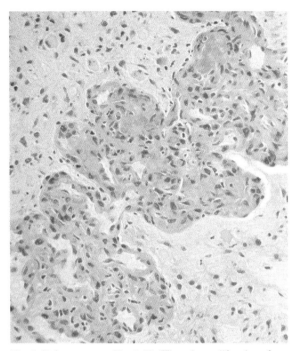

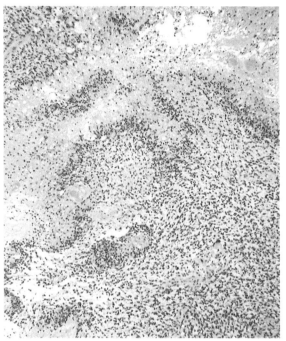

Fig. 2.51 Same case as Fig. 2.49. When the proliferation of endothelium is as disordered as this stasis and thrombosis are extremely common. CP HE × 205

Fig. 2.53 Same tissue as Fig. 2.52. The distinction between necrotic and viable tumour becomes much clearer after paraffin processing. CP HE × 80

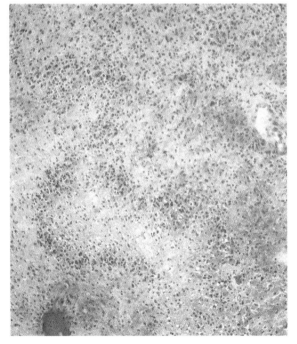

Fig. 2.52 Parietal glioblastoma. (M 28) The more darkly stained zone of nuclei bordering an area of necrosis is best appreciated at low magnification. CS HE × 80

Malignant gliomas involve the meninges more commonly than is usually appreciated, and may excite a fibroblastic reaction (Figs. 2.54–2.56) of such a degree that the tumour may clinically mimic a sarcoma or meningioma. A mesenchymal component may also develop de-novo from undifferentiated cells associated with proliferating blood vessels. In both circumstances the glial nature of the tumour may only be appreciated by examining several areas, especially those furthest from the superficial, more fibrous, portion. Staining for reticulin (Fig. 2.57) may demonstrate the perivascular origins of the proliferating fibroblasts and contrasts with the islands of glial tumour demonstrated in sections stained for GFAP (Fig. 2.58). Occasionally necrotic tumour evokes a similar focal fibrosis resulting in distortion of the local architecture termed a tertiary structure (Fig. 2.59). When the mesenchymal element is histologically malignant (Fig. 2.60) (usually a fibrosarcoma or an angiosarcoma, but sometimes mixed), the tumour is considered as a mixed glioblastoma-sarcoma to which the term gliosarcoma is sometimes applied.

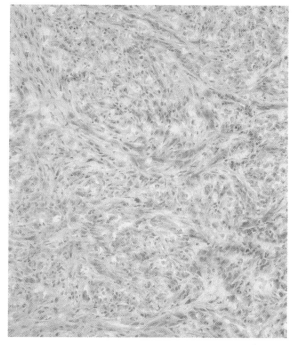

Fig. 2.55 Same case as Fig. 2.54. Infiltrating tumour cells are so compressed by proliferating mesenchymal cells that their glial nature is not obvious. CS HE × 128

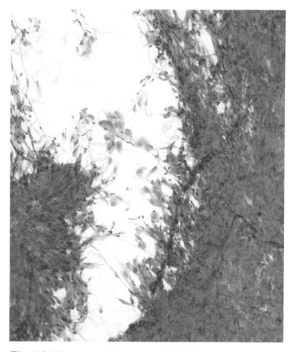

Fig. 2.54 Temporal glioblastoma. (M 57) Although clinically diagnosed as a meningioma neoplastic glial cells can be found amongst reactive fibrous tissue. SP HE × 128

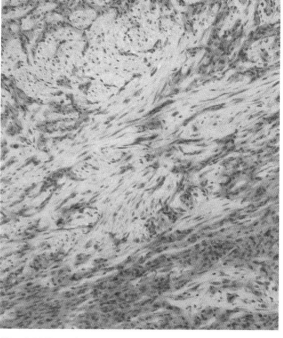

Fig. 2.56 Same tissue as the case in Fig. 2.54. After paraffin processing the tumour cells still bear little resemblance to a typical glioblastoma. CP HE × 128

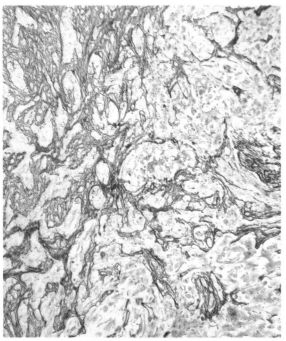

Fig. 2.57 Parietal glioblastoma. (M 44) This shows the junctional zone between the glioblastoma (right) and proliferating mesenchymal cells (left). PS RETIC × 80

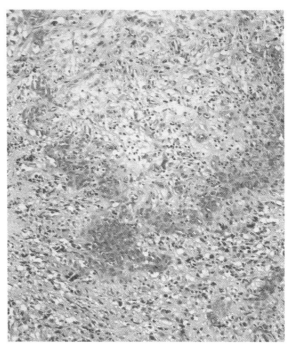

Fig. 2.59 Temporal glioblastoma. (M 71) Fibrosis (top) has developed in an area of necrosis separated from viable tumour by proliferating vessels. PS HE × 128

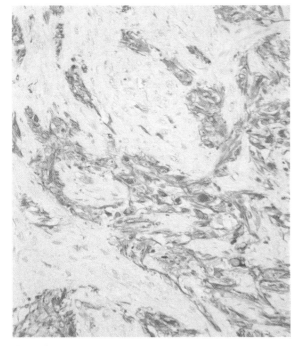

Fig. 2.58 Same case as Fig. 2.57. The malignant glial elements can be distinguished by their GFAP content from reactive fibroblasts. PS IP × 128

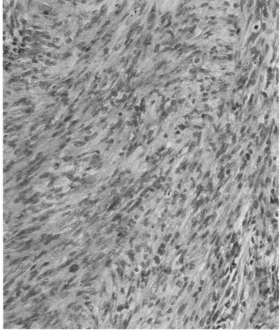

Fig. 2.60 Parasagittal glioblastoma—fibrosarcoma. (F 72) Tumour-related mesenchyme has sarcomatous features of high cellularity and mitotic rate. PS HE × 205

The range of appearances encompassed by the term glioblastoma includes small cell variants (Figs. 2.61–2.63) which must be distinguished from oat-cell carcinoma or primitive neuroectodermal tumour (PNET) (Ch. 4), spindle cell forms (Figs. 2.64 & 2.65) resembling sarcomas, giant cell forms (Figs. 2.66 & 2.67) and variants resembling epithelial cells (Figs. 2.68–2.70). The small cell variant (Figs. 2.61–2.63) lacks the tendency to form cell clusters that is typical of oat cell (and other) carcinomas (Figs. 14.2 & 14.3), and the malignant cells usually demonstrate some residual process formation, although this, however, may only become apparent on paraffin sections. Spindle cell morphology (Fig. 2.64) is usually a focal feature, but when it is the dominant pattern in a small biopsy there may be a resemblance to a sarcoma, an effect heightened in a paraffin section (Fig. 2.65) by a fascicular growth pattern. Smears from such a tumour will usually contain areas with more typical glial characteristics, and examination of further paraffin sections should reveal areas in which a glial nature is more obvious.

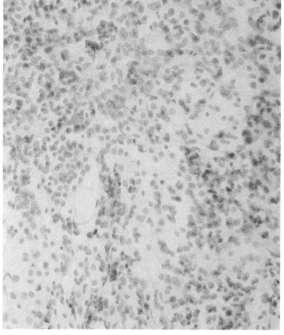

Fig. 2.62 Same case as Fig. 2.61. Diligent searching in such a tumour may reveal occasional cells with more typical astroglial features. SP HE × 205

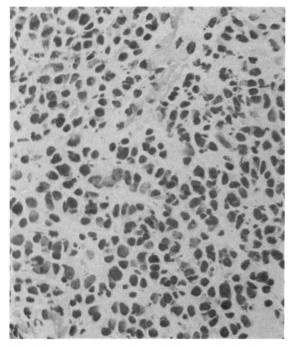

Fig. 2.61 Cervical cord small cell glioblastoma. (F 38) The appearances in this section resemble a PNET or anaplastic carcinoma. CS HE × 320

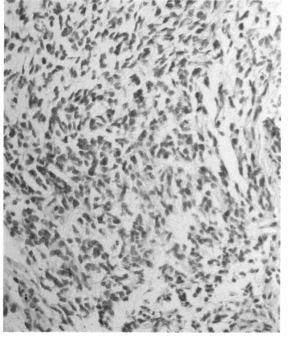

Fig. 2.63 Same case as Fig. 2.61. Paraffin processing reveals some cells with eosinophilic cytoplasm and scanty processes which betray their true nature. P HE × 205

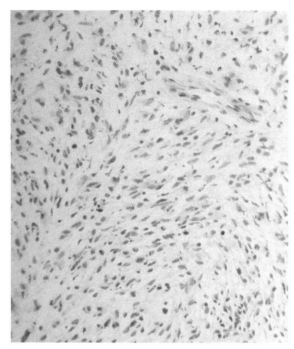

Fig. 2.64 Parietal glioblastoma. (M 50) Many cells have a spindle shape but cytoplasmic eosinophilia and processes identify an astroglial tumour. CS HE × 205

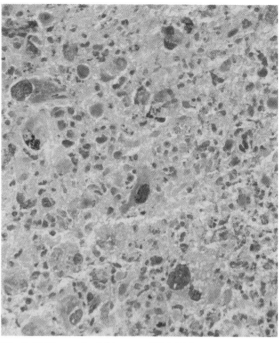

Fig. 2.66 Giant cell glioblastoma. (M 37) The giant cells stand out against a background of smaller, but clearly malignant, glial cells. CS HE × 205

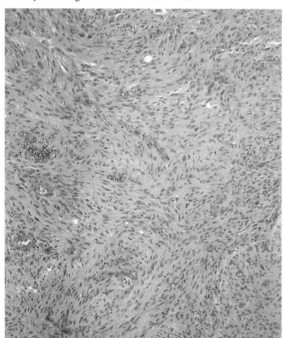

Fig. 2.65 Frontal glioblastoma. (M 61) A fascicular growth pattern may be more pronounced in paraffin sections. PS HE × 80

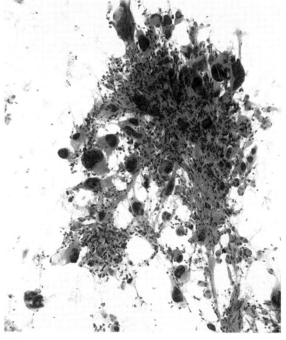

Fig. 2.67 Same case as Fig. 2.66. Although they are the most conspicuous feature the giant cells may be a relatively small proportion of the total. SP HE × 80

Where the tumour cells have lost the property of process formation, smears may show the clear cell margins, single cell separation and even clump formation more typically associated with epithelial tumours (Fig. 2.68). Further sampling may reveal areas with a more recognisably glioblastomatous appearance and examination of the infiltrating edge (if represented) will show a pattern of diffuse single cell infiltration rather than the clear boundary that characterises metastatic carcinoma. Where difficulty persists in paraffin sections (Fig. 2.69), and in other variants of glioblastoma described earlier, recourse to the immunohistochemical demonstration of GFAP may be necessary (Fig. 2.70). Although the presence of GFAP in this context is a clear indicator that the tumour is glial, the expression of GFAP by malignant astroglial tumours is neither inevitable nor by any means uniform within an individual lesion. In some cases vimentin is the main intermediate filament present. A GFAP-negative tumour with glial features should be examined carefully in several areas before concluding that it is not of astrocytic origin.

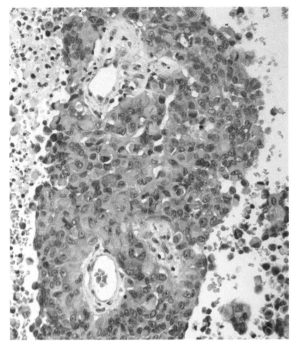

Fig. 2.69 Same case as Fig. 2.68. Sheets of cells clearly demarcated from areas of necrosis bear a close resemblance to a carcinoma. PS HE × 205

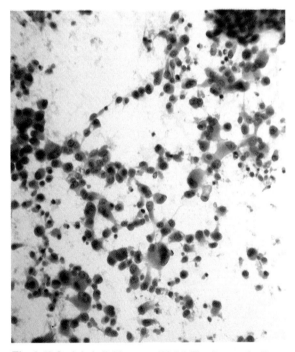

Fig. 2.68 Occipital glioblastoma. (M 34) The degree of cell separation and the paucity of cell processes is quite unlike typical glioblastomas. SP HE × 205

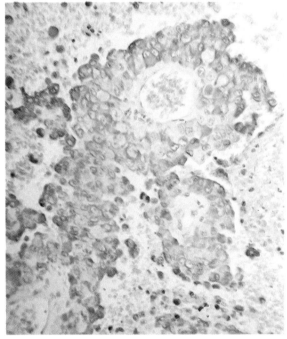

Fig. 2.70 Same case as Fig. 2.68. The expression by tumour cells of GFAP provides evidence that they are of an intrinsic astroglial nature. PS IP × 205

FURTHER READING

Barnard RO, Bradford R, Scott T, Thomas DGT 1986 Gliomyosarcoma. Report of a case of rhabdomyosarcoma arising in a malignant glioma. Acta Neuropathologica (Berlin) 69:23–27

Burger PC, Green SB 1987 Patient age, histologic features, and length of survival in patients with glioblastoma multiforme. Cancer 59:1617–1625

Burger PC, Vogel FS, Green SB, Strike TA 1985 Glioblastoma multiforme and anaplastic astrocytoma. Pathologic criteria and prognostic implications. Cancer 56:1106–1111

Burger PC, Vollmer RT 1980 Histologic factors of prognostic significance in the glioblastoma multiforme. Cancer 46:1179–1186

Ehrenreich T, Devlin JF 1958 A complex of glioblastoma and spindle-cell sarcoma with pulmonary metastasis. Archives of Pathology 66:536–549

Galloway PG, Roessman U 1986 Anaplastic astrocytoma mimicking metastatic carcinoma. American Journal of Surgical Pathology 10:728–732

Kishikawa M, Tsuda N, Fujii H, Nishimori I, Yokohama H, Kihara M 1986 Glioblastoma with sarcomatous component associated with myxoid change. A histochemical, immunohistochemical and electron microscopic study. Acta Neuropathologica (Berlin) 70:44–52

Kornfeld M 1986 Granular cell glioblastoma: a malignant granular cell neoplasm of astrocytic origin. Journal of Neuropathology and Experimental Neurology 45:447–462

Slowik F, Jellinger K, Gaszo L, Fischer J 1985 Gliosarcomas:Histological, immunohistochemical, ultrastructural, and tissue culture studies. Acta Neuropathologica (Berlin) 67:201–210

NOTES

Oligodendrogliomas most usually occur in the cerebral hemispheres and are generally reputed to be slowly growing with a favourable prognosis. Several large series have, however, shown that this is often not the case and tumours may show the rapid progression of a malignant lesion, sometimes with CSF spread.

The component cells are relatively regular in size and shape, with scanty eosinophilic cytoplasm which in smears may appear polar in distribution (Figs. 2.71 & 2.72). Cytoplasmic processes are not a feature of the parenchymal cell but the presence of astrocytes within the tumour (Fig. 2.71) should be appreciated and not lead to the diagnosis of an astroglial tumour.

Depending on the arrangement and density of blood vessels the tumour cells may occur in 'packets' enclosed in vascular elements (Fig. 2.72), or in sheets with inconspicuous vasculature (Fig. 2.73). The sparse cytoplasm, defined cell boundaries and vasculature may resemble a pituitary adenoma (p. 104) on cryostat sections (Fig. 2.74). Mitoses are variable in number and although necrosis is not common it may occur and, in the context of a frozen section where anisocytosis is exaggerated, this may lead to a diagnosis of malignant astrocytoma or glioblastoma. This problem is compounded by the fact that vascular proliferation is not unknown in oligodendrogliomas although the features of the cells in smears will help to distinguish them from other tumours.

Cellular shrinkage following processing results in perinuclear haloes (Fig. 2.75 & 2.76) which are not seen in smears (Figs. 2.71 & 2.72) or cryostat sections (Figs. 2.73 & 2.74). This effect is exaggerated when stellate fibrous astrocytes are scattered diffusely through the tumour, the processes tending to enclose individual cells which shrink away during processing. When the cells are surrounded by neuropil, as in an infiltrating edge, a similar phenomenon may occur, but is much less consistent so that a mixed picture of infiltrating small cells with, or without, haloes may result. Very similar appearances may be seen at the edge of other glial tumours (Fig. 2.10) and in these circumstances are not diagnostic of oligodendroglioma (p. 10).

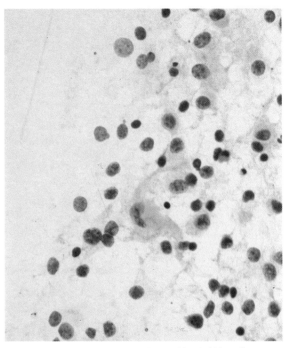

Fig. 2.71 Frontal oligodendroglioma. (M 61) Although most tumour cells have scanty cytoplasm and few processes, astrocytes can usually be found in smears. SP HE × 400

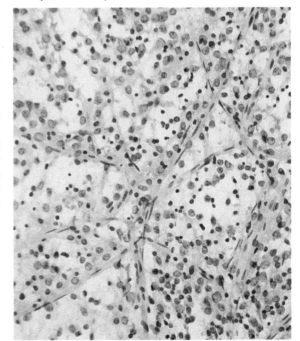

Fig. 2.72 Frontal oligodendroglioma. (F 50) Tumour cells, most with little cytoplasm, are enclosed by a fine vascular network. SP HE × 205

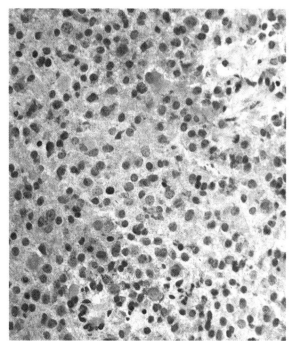

Fig. 2.73 Frontal oligodendroglioma. (F 27) The separation of cells reflects the paucity of process formation which contrasts with that of an astrocyte (top). CS HE × 320

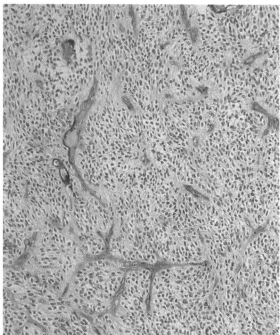

Fig. 2.75 Occipital oligodendroglioma. (M 5) A fine vascular framework, calcified in places, encloses cells showing the effects of shrinkage. PS HE × 128

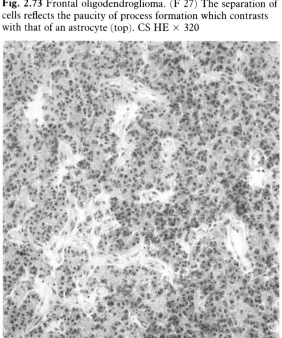

Fig. 2.74 Parietal oligodendroglioma. (M 38) The absence of artefactual haloes in cryostat sections may result in a misdiagnosis of pituitary adenoma. CS HE × 128

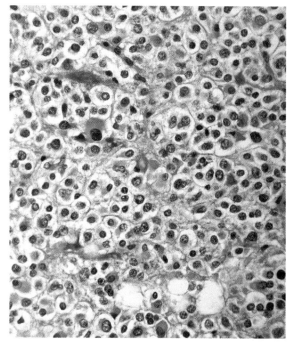

Fig. 2.76 Frontal oligodendroglioma. (M 55) Although most cells consist of a nucleus in an empty space some do have eosinophilic cytoplasm. PS HE × 320

One feature of oligodendrogliomas that may lead to their being suspected clinically is the presence of calcification. This is often dense, and may occur both in the tumour and in adjacent brain which may also be gliotic. This calcium deposition, which may be massive, frequently occurs in relation to blood vessels (Fig. 2.77). Although common in oligodendrogliomas, calcification is not inevitable and it should be remembered that similar degrees of calcification may occur in astrocytomas (Fig. 2.22).

Staining oligodendrogliomas for GFAP will usually reveal one of two patterns of expression. Cells with the appearance of normal fibrous astrocytes may be seen, sometimes in considerable numbers, contrasting with unstained tumour cells (Fig. 2.78). Distinct from what may be structural astrocytes, cells expressing GFAP may constitute a significant proportion of the parenchyma of tumours with a typical oligodendroglial pattern (Fig. 2.79). It is important to recognise these tumours as oligodendrogliomas rather than astrocytomas despite the expression of what is more usually considered to be a marker of astrocytes, although it is not yet clear whether this expression is of any prognostic value. There is clear evidence that the conventional markers of malignancy in astrocytic tumours (necrosis, mitotic activity and vascular proliferation) do have a bearing on subsequent behaviour and should be taken into account. Nevertheless there is, as yet, no agreement as to what constitute histological criteria for applying the term malignant to an oligodendroglioma.

Within otherwise typical tumours areas may be seen in which cells without haloes show quite different arrangements. These include palisading (Fig. 2.80), a trabecular architecture (Fig. 2.81), or cellular clustering, the latter resembling the pattern seen in some astrocytomas (Figs. 2.23–2.25). Rarely mucin may accumulate intra- or extracellularly. Where an oligodendroglioma contains areas of tumour with the architecture and cytology of an astrocytoma the lesion should be diagnosed as an oligoastrocytoma (Fig. 2.82), although the relationship between the cells comprising oligodendrogliomas and astrocytomas is by no means clear.

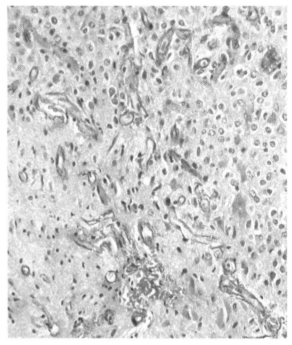

Fig. 2.77 Frontal oligodendroglioma. (F 51) Calcification in this tumour is predominantly in vessel walls but in other cases may be interstitial. PS HE × 205

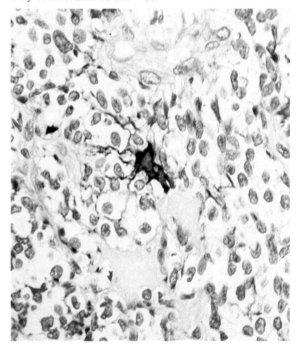

Fig. 2.78 Occipital oligodendroglioma. (M 5) (same case as Fig. 2.75) A process-forming astrocyte containing GFAP contrasts with non-staining tumour cells. PS IP × 512

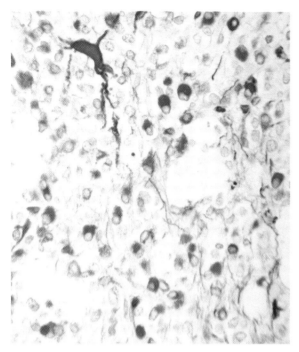

Fig. 2.79 Frontal oligodendroglioma. (M 55) (same case as Fig. 2.76) Many tumour cells contain GFAP but are distinct from process-forming astrocytes. PS IP × 320

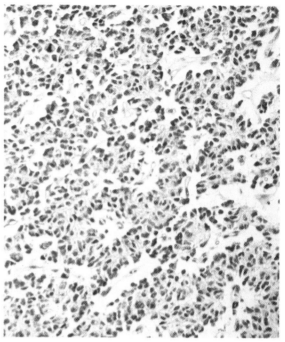

Fig. 2.81 Frontal oligodendroglioma. (M 51) A trabecular pattern results when perinuclear halo development is minimal. PS HE × 205

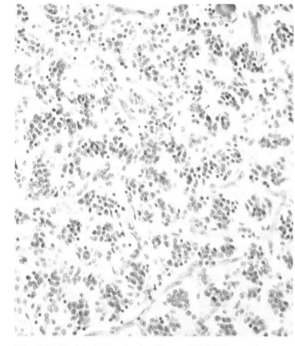

Fig. 2.80 Occipital oligodendroglioma. (M 2) The regular alignment of cells within a vascular network in this tumour results in a palisaded appearance. PS HE × 205

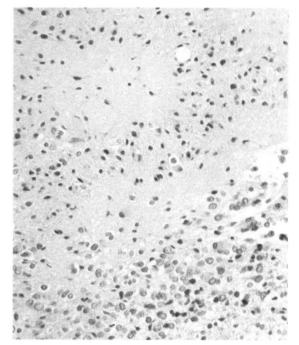

Fig. 2.82 Frontal oligoastrocytoma. (F 38) Oligodendroglial cells (below) contrast with process-forming astrocytic elements (above). PS HE × 205

FURTHER READING

Burger PC, Rawlings CE, Cox EB, McLendon RE, Schold SC, Bullard DE 1987 Clinicopathologic correlations in the oligodendroglioma. Cancer 59:1345–1352

Hart MN, Petito CK, Earle KM 1974 Mixed gliomas. Cancer 33:134–140

Herpers MJHM, Budka H 1984 Glial fibrillary acidic protein (GFAP) in oligodendroglial tumours: gliofibrillary oligodendroglioma and transitional oligoastrocytoma as subtypes of oligodendroglioma. Acta Neuropathologica (Berlin) 64:265–272

Ludwig Cl, Smith MT, Godfrey AD, Armbrustmacher VW 1986 A clinicopathological study of 323 patients with oligodendrogliomas. Annals of Neurology 19:15–21

Mork SJ, Halvorsen TB, Lindegaard K-F, Eide GE 1986 Oligodendroglioma. Histologic evaluation and prognosis. Journal of Neuropathology and Experimental Neurology 45:65–78

Mork SJ, Lindegaard K-F, Halvorsen TB, Lehmann EH, Solgaard T, Hatlevoll R, Harvei S, Ganz J 1985 Oligodendroglioma: incidence and biological behavior in a defined population. Journal of Neurosurgery 63:881–889

Nakagawa Y, Perentes E, Rubinstein LG 1986 Immunohistochemical characterization of oligodendrogliomas: an analysis of multiple markers. Acta Neuropathologica (Berlin) 72:15–22

Smith MT, Ludwig Cl, Godfrey AD, Armbrustmacher VW 1983 Grading of oligodendrogliomas. Cancer 52:2107–2114

Wilkinson IMS, Anderson JR, Holmes AE 1987 Oligodendroglioma: an analysis of 42 cases. Journal of Neurology, Neurosurgery and Psychiatry 50:304–312.

NOTES

Although it is most commonly encountered in the fourth ventricle the ependymoma can arise from the ependymal cells of any ventricle, the spinal canal (almost always in adults) or the filum terminale. Ependymal cells are normally found lining the ventricles and, in smaller numbers, in the subependymal zone. Areas reminiscent of both locations are found in ependymal neoplasia.

A basic primary tumour structure exists but the appearances of biopsy samples can vary considerably depending on the area of the tumour biopsied. In addition variations or modifications of this basic pattern result in two defined variants—the subependymoma and the myxopapillary ependymoma.

It is important to recognise that the component cells form different structures depending on whether they are forming a surface (as in a ventricular lining) or whether they are mixed with astroglial-like elements that may not be neoplastic (as in normal subependymal tissue). Variations that are seen in ependymomas can therefore be interpreted as the result of varying admixtures of neoplastic ependymal cells and structural astroglial elements.

The surface-lining properties of ependymal cells are manifest as tubules, clefts or small papillae (Figs. 2.83 & 2.84). Since their visualisation depends on correct orientation these are more readily seen in tissue sections than smear preparations, although in cryostat sections they are seldom prominent. Ependymal lined clefts may develop as a result of invagination or inclusion of reactive non-neoplastic ependyma overlying a primary astrocytic tumour, and other more typical primary structure must be sought to substantiate the diagnosis of an ependymoma.

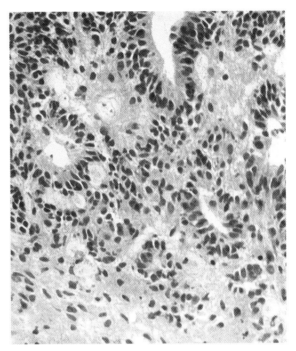

Fig. 2.83 Fourth ventricle ependymoma. (M 4) In this superficial biopsy ependymal cells form tubules and clefts with intervening fibrillary matrix. CS HE × 320

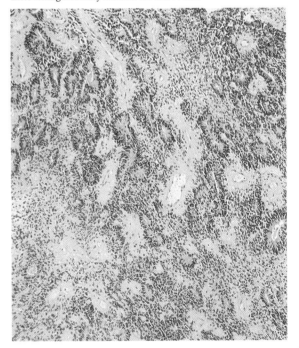

Fig. 2.84 Same tissue as Fig. 2.83 A tubular pattern is usually only prominent towards the tumour surface (top) where small papillae may occasionally be seen. PS HE × 80

The archetypal primary structure that characterises an ependymoma results from the perivascular orientation of tumour cells with supporting astroglial-like elements. These gliovascular structures are responsible for the retention of tumour cells around vessels and the resulting papillary appearance of smears (Fig. 2.85). They also give rise to the characteristic fibrillary perivascular zone that separates tumour cell bodies and nuclei from vessels (Figs. 2.86 & 2.87). The distinction between ependymal cells and fibrillary astroglial-like elements can be emphasised by staining for GFAP, but the pattern is usually sufficiently distinctive on H & E sections.

Cytologically the cells are relatively small and uniform, with visible cytoplasm on smears (Fig. 2.85) and may resemble the component cells of an oligodendroglioma. The absence of the fine capillary network that characterises the latter (Fig. 2.72), and the presence of gliovascular structures, should aid in their distinction.

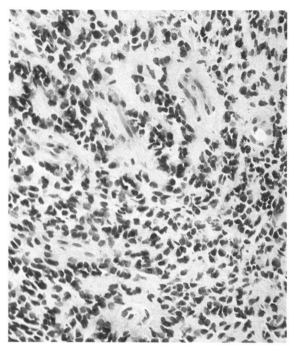

Fig. 2.86 Fourth ventricle ependymoma. (M 8) In deeper areas of the tumour the cells are separated from small vessels by an intervening fibrillary zone. CS HE × 205

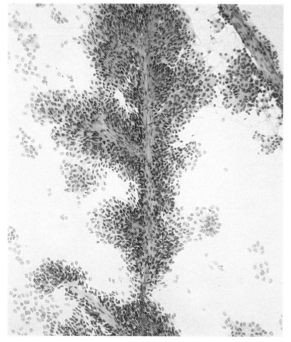

Fig. 2.85 Fourth ventricle ependymoma. (F 60) In this smear the adherence of cells around blood vessels and the lack of pleomorphism is well seen. SP HE × 80

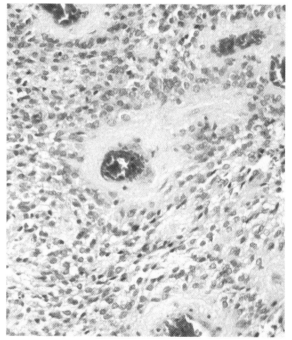

Fig. 2.87 Same case as Fig. 2.86. Fixation enhances the contrast between the fibrillar perivascular zones and surrounding cellular areas. PS HE × 205

Elongated cells with prominent processes may be seen in relation to blood vessels in smears (Fig. 2.88), emphasising both the astroglial-like component of the gliovascular structures, and the need to recognise that cells with astroglial features occur in ependymal tumours. Indeed some spinal ependymomas which show a predominance of astroglial-like elements (and so resemble pilocytic astrocytomas) have been held to represent a tumour expressing the characteristics of the primitive ependymoglial precursor cell (tanycyte) of the developing brain. A misdiagnosis of astrocytoma in more typical ependymomas will be avoided by recognition of the typical perivascular arrangement of the ependymal elements. This error is more likely to occur if the biopsy derives from the interface zone between normal brain and tumour.

The neoplastic ependymal cells infiltrate beyond the macroscopic margins of the tumour in small numbers and therefore do not show the typical primary perivascular arrangement of an ependymoma (Fig. 2.89). The dominance of astroglial elements (whose increased numbers may be a reaction to the neoplasm) may make a correct diagnosis difficult. If there is a strong clinical suspicion at operation that the tumour is ependymal assurance should be sought that the biopsy under study has derived from superficial or primary structure rather than tumour/brain interface before an ependymoma is excluded. Similar appearances may be encountered in a subependymona (p. 45) which should also be considered as a differential diagnosis.

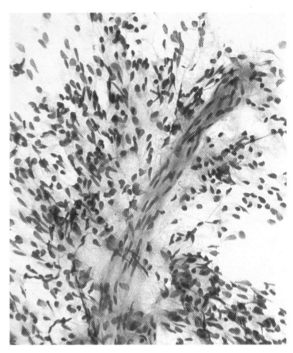

Fig. 2.88 Fourth ventricle ependymoma. (M 6) The structure of the perivascular zone is reflected in the mixture of astrocyte-like and ependymal cells. SP HE × 205

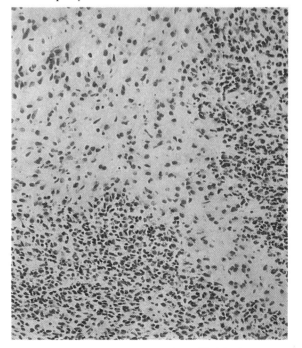

Fig. 2.89 Fourth ventricle ependymoma. (M 8) At the tumour edge the primary structure is less apparent and adjacent astrocytes (top) are increased in number. CS HE × 128

The infiltration of neoplastic cells beyond the macroscopic margins of the tumour is partly responsible for the risk of recurrence in ependymomas, but true malignancy is rare. When it occurs the primary structure is usually retained allowing recognition of an ependymal nature. Necrosis, high cellularity and mitoses (rare in ordinary ependymomas) indicate a malignant lesion (Figs. 2.90 & 2.91), and although there is a correlation with a poorer prognosis histology is not a good predictor for the individual patient. Distinction should be made from a primitive neuro-ectodermal tumour (PNET) with ependymal differentiation (the so-called ependymoblastoma). This tumour is composed entirely of primitive cells and, although a perivascular arrangement may be seen, the typical fibrillary component is lacking. Where tubules form they are lined by dividing primitive cells (Fig. 2.92), but frequently other forms of differentiation (astrocytic or oligodendroglial) may be apparent and pure tumours of primitive ependymal cells are rare.

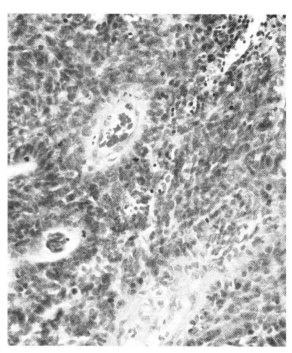

Fig. 2.91 Same case as Fig. 2.90. High cell density, mitoses and necrosis characterise the malignant ependymoma although the basic pattern remains. PS HE × 205

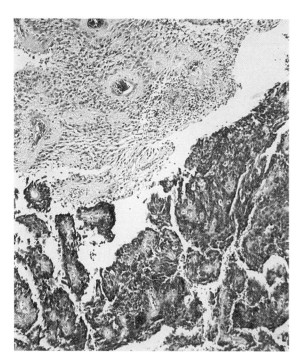

Fig. 2.90 Fourth ventricle ependymoma. (M 8) Typical tumour (above) contrasts with an area of malignancy in which a residual primary structure is visible. PS HE × 80

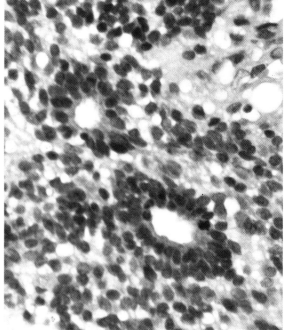

Fig. 2.92 Cerebral primitive neuroectodermal tumour. (M 6) Ependymoblastic tubules are formed by primitive cells that also form the rest of the tumour. PS HE × 512

The subependymoma is best interpreted as the result of a predominance of astroglial elements in a lesion of primarily ependymal origin, although some consider that it arises from a distinct subependymal cell and histological similarities with some astrocytomas (Figs. 2.17–2.20) may indicate a common origin. It is not commonly encountered as a clinical problem, and has a poorer prognosis when forming a mixed tumour associated with areas of typical ependymoma. The picture is a distortion of the typical structure of an ependymoma in that the tumour cells are more dispersed and do not show the same degree of perivascular orientation (Figs. 2.93 & 2.94). There are much larger areas of gliofibrillary matrix, within which calcium deposition may occur (Fig. 2.95), with varying numbers of ependymal cells which only form characteristic primary structure in areas of high density.

Distinction from a low grade astrocytoma or the edge of an ependymoma will depend on adequate and representative sampling but caution should be exercised with small biopsies and if necessary a firm opinion deferred until paraffin sections are available.

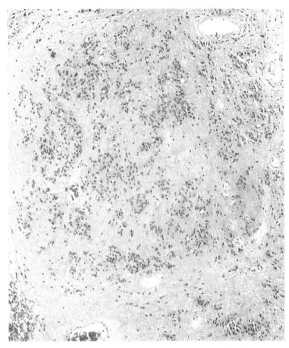

Fig. 2.94 Fourth ventricle subependymoma. (M 55) The dispersal of the ependymal elements is better appreciated at lower magnification. PS HE × 80

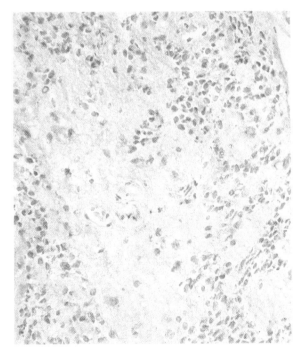

Fig. 2.93 Fourth ventricle subependymoma. (M 53) A prominent gliofibrillary matrix separates the ependymal cells and causes resemblance to an astrocytoma. CS HE × 205

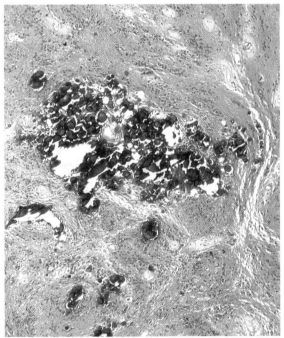

Fig. 2.95 Same case as Fig. 2.94. Calcification, a predominant fibrillary matrix and inconspicuous ependymal cells are typical features. PS HE × 64

This distinctive tumour typically occurs in the region of the filum terminale, but may be found higher up the spinal cord or even in the overlying subcutaneous tissue. In the subarachnoid space it is a loosely structured lesion which, although frequently encapsulated by meninges, diffusely surrounds spinal nerve roots and the cauda equina. In essence it is a primary ependymal neoplasm whose basic architecture is altered by a characteristic response of the mesenchymal component of the blood vessels around which it grows.

Retention of the typical ependymomatous primary structure is seen in the papillary pattern of the smear and the cytology of the component cells (Fig. 2.96). Areas of more solid tumour with the characteristic perivascular orientation of cerebral ependymomas may be found, especially in lesions proximal to the cauda equina.

The accumulation of mucins within the perivascular connective tissue sheath (beneath the basement membrane upon which the tumour cells rest) leads first to distension of cell masses and then to the separation of small blebs of mucin, with surrounding cells (Figs. 2.97 & 2.98), which form cysts or papillae. Staining with toluidine blue (Fig. 2.99) demonstrates the relationship of the neoplastic glial cells to these pools of metachromatic mucin which may show only faint basophilic staining in H & E preparations.

Progressive distension and disruption of primary structure results in the typical myxopapillary appearance (Figs. 2.100–2.101). Failure to recognise that most of the larger mucin-filled cysts enclosed by tumour cells are centered on blood vessels, combined with the mild anisocytosis seen on cryostat sections, may lead to a diagnosis of metastatic adenocarcinoma. The smear appearances, however, indicate quite clearly (especially when solid areas of tumour are available for examination) that cytologically the cells are ependymal, or at least glial, and not epithelial.

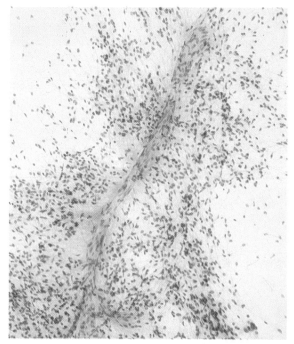

Fig. 2.96 Lumbar myxopapillary ependymoma. (M 19) The vascular orientation and cytology of the tumour reflects its glial and ependymal nature. SP HE × 80

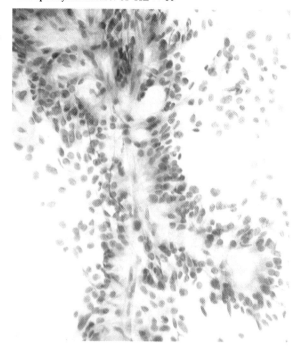

Fig. 2.97 Same case as Fig. 2.96. Small collections of mucin separate tumour cell clumps from subjacent blood vessels. SP HE × 205

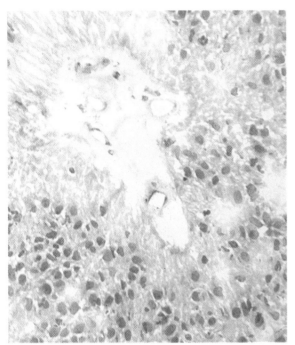

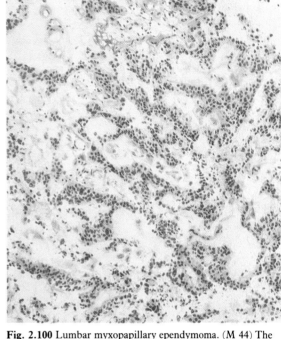

Fig. 2.98 Same case as Fig. 2.96. The ependymal appearance of the cells and the perivascular separation by mucin are better seen in this section. CS HE × 256

Fig. 2.100 Lumbar myxopapillary ependymoma. (M 44) The resemblance to adenocarcinoma is belied by the presence of vessels within the 'acini'. CS HE × 80

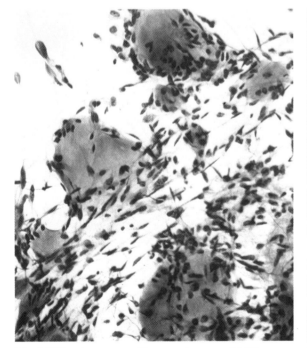

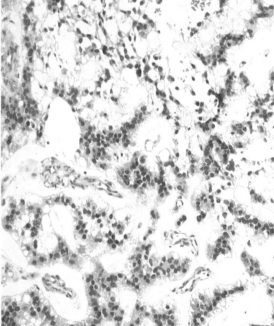

Fig. 2.99 Lumbar myxopapillary ependymoma. (M 48) Toluidine blue staining reveals metachromatic mucin blebs enclosed by tumour cells. SP TOL B × 205

Fig. 2.101 Same case as Fig. 2.100. After paraffin processing the relationship of tumour cells to blood vessels and the intervening mucin is much clearer. PS HE × 128

The accumulation of mucins around blood vessels weakens their structure with the result that haemorrhage is common (Fig. 2.102). Tertiary structure with scarring and enclosure of cells may be difficult to distinguish from invasion (Fig. 2.103). Even when there is genuine invasion by tumour cells this does not appear to correlate with the risk of recurrence which is more related to the degree of circumscription of the tumour and the completeness of surgical removal. Cytological atypia is rare but may be found in subsequent paraffin sections (Fig. 2.104). As with invasion there is no clear correlation with outcome.

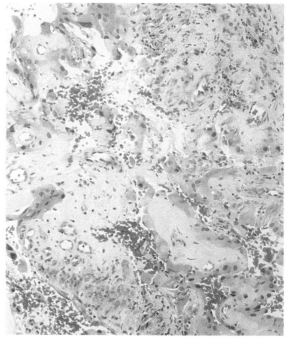

Fig. 2.103 Same case as Fig. 2.102. Scarring by reactive fibrous tissue further distorts the tumour pattern and the entrapment of cells resembles invasion. PS HE × 128

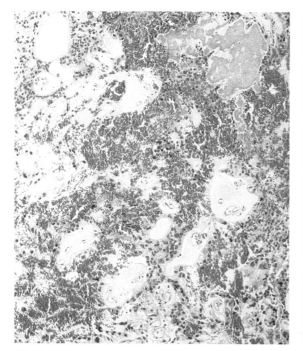

Fig. 2.102 Lumbar myxopapillary ependymoma. (M 44) Haemorrhage distorts the tumour structure and provides a stimulus for fibrous scarring. PS HE × 80

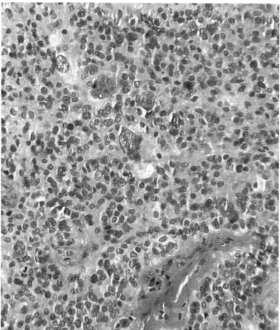

Fig. 2.104 Same case as Fig. 2.102. The enlarged atypical nuclei (here in a more typically ependymomatous area) are without significance for tumour behaviour. PS HE × 205

FURTHER READING

Azarelli B, Rekate HL, Roessmann U 1977 Subependymoma. A case report with ultrastructural study. Acta Neuropathologica (Berlin) 40:279–282

Friede RL, Pollak A 1978 The cytogenetic basis for classifying ependymomas. Journal of Neuropathology and Experimental Neurology 37:103–118

Helwig EB, Stern JB 1984 Subcutaneous sacrococcygeal myxopapillary ependymoma. A clinicopathologic study of 32 cases. American Journal of Clinical Pathology 81:156–161

Ilgren EB, Stiller CA, Hughes JT, Silberman D, Steckel N, Kaye A 1984 Ependymomas: a clinical and pathologic study Part II—survival features. Clinical Neuropathology 3:122–127

Jooma R, Torrens MJ, Bradshaw J, Brownell B 1985 Subependymomas of the fourth ventricle. Journal of Neurosurgery 62:508–512

Mork SJ, Loken AC 1977 Ependymoma: a follow-up study of 101 cases. Cancer 40:907–915

Mork SJ, Rubinstein LJ 1985 Ependymoblastoma. A reappraisal of a rare embryonic tumor. Cancer 55:1536–1542

Sonneland PRL, Scheithauer BW, Onofrio B 1985 Myxopapillary ependymoma. A clinicopathologic and immunocytochemical study of 77 cases. Cancer 56:883–893

West CR, Bruce DA, Duffner PK 1985 Ependymomas. Factors in clinical and diagnostic staging. Cancer 56:1812–1816

NOTES

The papilloma is a relatively rare lesion of the choroid plexus epithelium, commoner in the fourth ventricle and in childhood, but also occurring in adults and in the lateral ventricles. Typically it causes a hydrocephalus, either by simple obstruction or excessive CSF production.

The appearances of a smear reflect the papillary nature of the lesion; numerous fine papillae are usually visible (Fig. 2.105) formed by a single layer of cuboidal or columnar epithelium over a fine fibrovascular core (Fig. 2.106) within which calcospherites may be found (as in normal choroid plexus) (Fig. 2.107). At the bases of fine peripheral papillae larger fibrovascular structures are seen and in these areas cross cutting of the bases of the clefts between papillae may give rise to the spurious appearance of invasion (Fig. 2.108). Cytological atypia is rare but if present in severe degree may raise the question of malignant change in a pre-existing papilloma. Irradiation of a benign lesion may also cause cytological change although mitoses would not be expected.

The component papillae may undergo cystic swelling due to accumulation of fluid within the stroma so that the fibrovascular cores become inconspicuous and the lesion appears to consist of epithelial cysts or tubules (Fig. 2.109) resembling a myxopapillary or papillary ependymoma. The smear reveals not fine papillae but sheets of the epithelial cells that are covering the distended fronds (Fig. 2.110) and at first sight these may be disconcerting in their similarity to the cell masses of an ependymoma (p. 42). Realisation that these are extreme examples of the fragments of covering epithelium and the numerous single cells that are seen in more typical lesions, should enable the correct diagnosis to be reached.

Rare examples of bilateral lesions do occur and in these circumstances a clear distinction between bilateral papillomas and papillary hyperplasia cannot really be made histologically. Their distinction will depend on whether there are discrete lesions or a diffuse increase in size of the choroid plexuses.

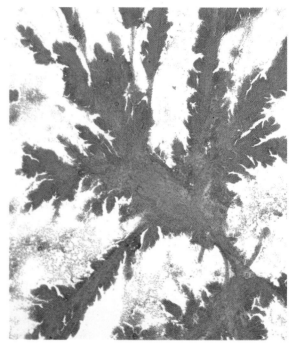

Fig. 2.105 Choroid plexus papilloma. (M 11) At low magnification the papillary arrangement of epithelium over vascular cores is easy to see. SP HE × 32

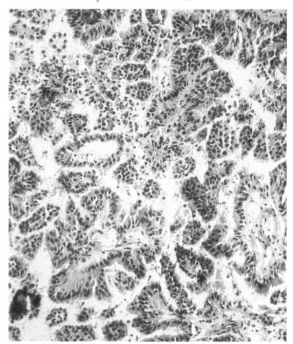

Fig. 2.106 Same case as Fig. 2.105. A layer of epithelium covers fine fibrovascular cores which contain scattered calcospherites. CS HE × 128

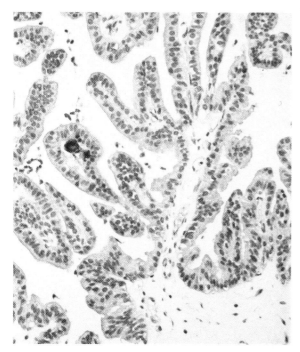

Fig. 2.107 Same as Fig. 2.105. The tumour epithelium closely resembles that of normal choroid although its arrangement is disordered. PS HE × 205

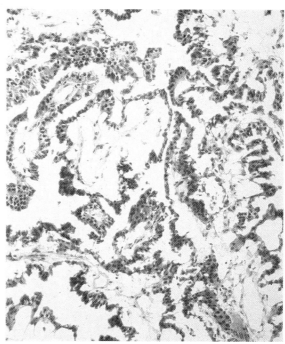

Fig. 2.109 Choroid plexus papilloma. (F 22) Fluid accumulation in the stromal cores masks the papillary nature of the tumour. CS HE × 128

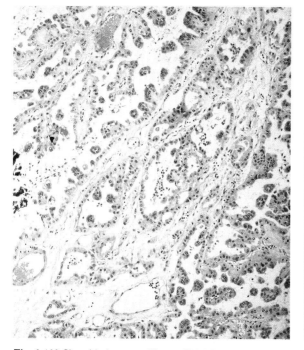

Fig. 2.108 Choroid plexus papilloma. (F 32) The appearance of invasion results from cross-cutting and there are no other features of malignancy. PS HE × 80

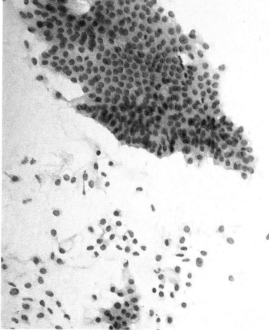

Fig. 2.110 Same case as Fig. 2.109. Epithelial sheets may be mistaken for solid tumour fragments if the separation of cells (bottom) is not recognised. SP HE × 205

The diagnosis of malignancy in a choroid plexus tumour should be based on the standard criteria of cytological atypia, mitotic activity and evidence of single cell infiltration into the fibrovascular cores. The definitive diagnosis of a primary choroid plexus carcinoma should, however, be made with extreme circumspection. The appearances of a malignant papillary carcinoma (Fig. 2.111), especially with calcospherites in a patient of appropriate age and sex, should first lead to the exclusion of a primary thyroid, ovarian or other adeno-carcinoma metastatic to the brain with involvement of choroid plexus. Only when such exclusion is certain can the diagnosis be confidently accepted, and this may require the passage of several years (Fig. 2.112). In children, or where there is known to have been a pre-existing benign papilloma, the diagnosis of primary choroid plexus malignancy may be made with more certainty.

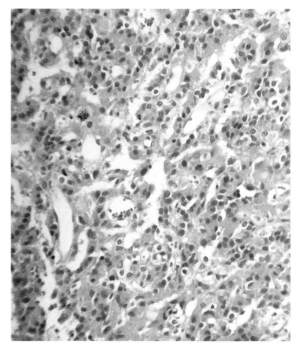

Fig. 2.111 Choroid plexus carcinoma. (M 47) This is a recurrence of a tumour diagnosed three years earlier as a metastatic adenopapillary carcinoma. PS HE × 205

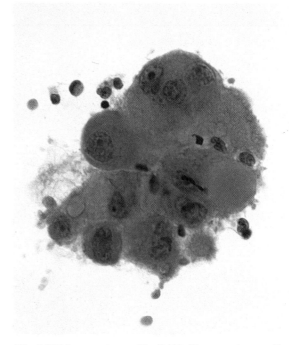

Fig. 2.112 Same patient as Fig. 2.111. Five years later malign-ant cells were widespread in the CSF with spinal deposits but no extraneural tumour was found. CYTO HE × 512

FURTHER READING

Ghatak NR, McWhorter JM 1976 Ultrastructural evidence for CSF production by a choroid plexus papilloma. Journal of Neurosurgery 45:409–415

McComb RD, Burger PC 1983 Choroid plexus carcinoma. Report of a case with immunohistochemical and ultrastructural observations. Cancer 51:470–475

Welch K, Strand R, Bresnan M, Cavazzuti V 1983 Congenital hydrocephalus due to villous hypertrophy of the telencephalic choroid plexuses. Journal of Neurosurgery 59:172–175

NOTES

3 MENINGEAL TUMOURS

The meningioma is the commonest extracerebral intracranial tumour and usually has a characteristic histological appearance but variant patterns are frequent and, on occasions, diagnostically taxing. It arises from the arachnoidal lining (meningothelial) cells but involves dural collagen so early that it becomes a lesion with a dural attachment.

Meningiomas have smooth lobulated outlines and (usually) a clear demarcation from adjacent brain (Fig. 3.1) which nonetheless may be deeply indented. Although frequently described as encapsulated they lack a true confining connective tissue capsule, and histologically the 'capsule' is usually composed of compressed meninges, sometimes with an adherent layer of gliotic superficial cortex. Commoner in adults than children, and in females than males, they are most frequent in the cranial cavities related to falx or cerebral convexities. Other well recognised sites are olfactory groove, optic foramen, sphenoid ridge, posterior fossa and lateral ventricle. In the spinal canal they are second in frequency to neurilemomas.

Whilst the brain is usually not invaded the tumour almost invariably infiltrates dura, frequently with venous invasion (Fig. 3.2), and may extend into subcutaneous tissue and bone (Figs. 3.3 & 3.4). Extension into bone is sometimes non-destructive, and an osteoblastic reaction with an overlying hyperostosis is frequent. Central necrosis is a feature of larger lesions and is probably the result of vascular insufficiency.

The arachnoidal cells that comprise meningiomas possess abundant intermediate filaments, mostly vimentin, widely interdigitated cell membranes and desmosomal cell junctions (Fig. 3.5). The interdigitation of cell processes results in a syncytial appearance in routine tissue sections and the term syncytial is used for the commonest histological pattern.

The reticulin pattern in meningiomas is coarse and irregular (Fig. 3.6) reflecting the distribution of collagen (some of which may be of dural origin) and is a useful distinguishing feature from neurilemomas which have a fine pericellular pattern (Fig. 5.11).

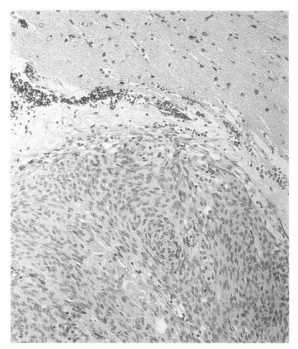

Fig. 3.1 Frontal meningioma. (F 76) A zone of compressed arachnoid separates tumour tissue (below) from indented cortex (above). PS HE × 128

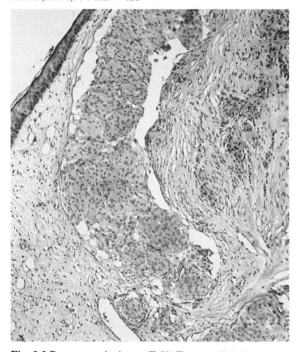

Fig. 3.2 Petrous meningioma. (F 53) Tumour clinically diagnosed as glomus jugulare paraganglioma lies in a small vein beneath the tympanic membrane . PS HE × 80

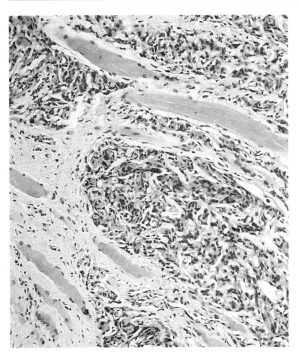

Fig. 3.3 Temporal meningioma. (M 52) Tumour infiltrates the temporalis muscle having extended through the squamous temporal bone. PS HE × 128

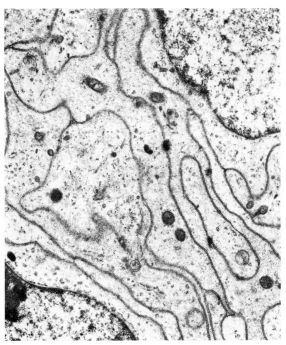

Fig. 3.5 Frontal meningioma. (M 43) Interdigitated cell processes with desmosomal cell junctions but without external lamina are typical features. EM × 14 500

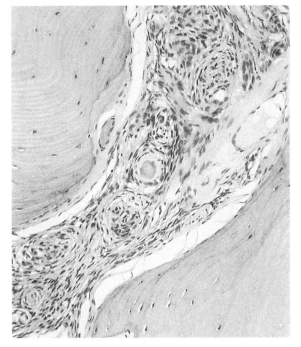

Fig. 3.4 Spinal meningioma. (F 55) Histologically typical tumour lies between bone trabeculae showing no osteoclastic or osteoblastic reaction. PS HE × 160

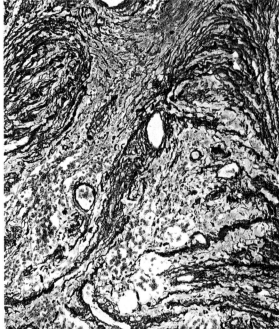

Fig. 3.6 Spinal meningioma. (M 80) Irregular distribution of collagen and the lack of regular pericellular basement membrane is apparent. PS RETIC × 128

In a typical syncytial meningioma the characteristics of the component cells, and their relations to each other, result in the presence of single cells and small cell groups in a smear (Fig. 3.7). The latter frequently form whorled or concentric clusters which are paralleled in the appearances of cryostat (Fig. 3.8) and paraffin (Fig. 3.9) sections. The uniformity of cell size and nuclear appearance is a striking feature, and although scattered large aberrant nuclei (Fig. 3.10) may be seen the pleomorphism and mitoses of a malignant epithelial tumour are lacking. Degenerative features such as intercellular oedema and xanthoma cell aggregates (Fig. 3.10) are usually focal and examination of other areas will reveal more typical appearances. Invaginations of cytoplasm into the nucleus give rise to eosinophilic pseudo-inclusions (Fig. 3.11) which, although characteristic, are neither inevitable nor specific.

Variant forms include psammomatous, angiomatous, fibroblastic, myxoid and 'clear cell' (due to intracellular glycogen); many tumours, however, show features transitional between one, or more, of these and a typical syncytial lesion and are referred to as transitional meningiomas. Secretory meningiomas prossess intracellular lumina which show cytokeratin and epithelial membrane antigen (EMA) expression and contain hyaline inclusions. In small biopsies from tumours that have infiltrated extensively (Fig. 3.2) these latter findings may suggest carcinoma, but the cytokeratin expression is focal rather than uniform.

These different histological types are without prognostic significance, although the atypical form (p. 64), in which mitoses, necrosis and cortical invasion occur, is associated with a higher risk of recurrence. Other major factors that have been implicated in the risk of recurrence include location of tumour (especially sphenoid ridge), extent of resection, multicentricity, patient age and sex. On rare occasions necrosis results in a focal or predominant papillary pattern (Fig. 3.12) consisting of a perivascular arrangement of tumour cells. Tumours with this feature have a higher incidence of recurrence and, more importantly, of metastasis.

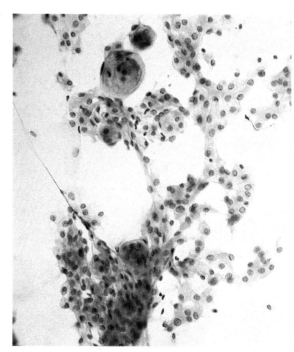

Fig. 3.7 Tentorial meningioma. (F 62) The uniformity of cell size, whorl formation and the easy separation of cells typify meningioma smears. SP HE × 205

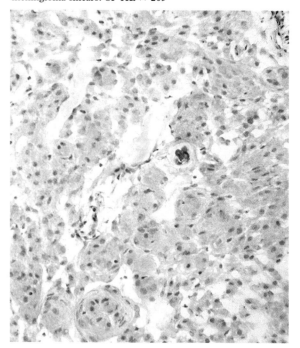

Fig. 3.8 Same case as Fig. 3.7. A cryostat section shows whorl formation with occasional calcifications (psammoma bodies) paralleling the smear features. CS HE × 205

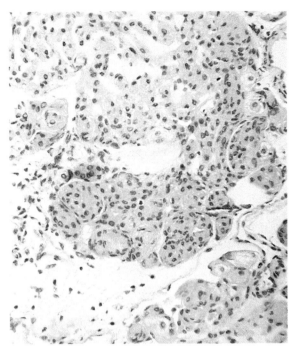

Fig. 3.9 Same tissue as Fig. 3.8. The mixture of whorl formation and areas of less defined architecture is common in syncytial meningiomas. CP HE × 205

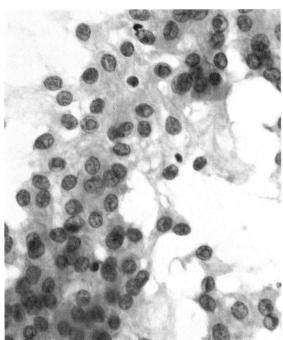

Fig. 3.11 Petrous meningioma. (F 46) Eosinophilic pseudo-inclusions in many tumour nuclei result from invaginations of cytoplasm. SP HE × 512

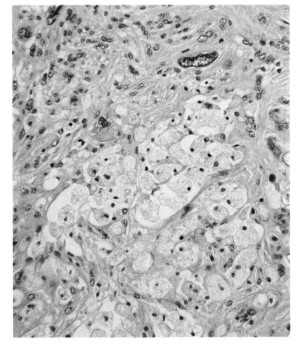

Fig. 3.10 Parietal meningioma. (M 56) Xanthoma cells and atypical nuclei may mimic a neurilemoma but are without prognostic significance. PS HE × 205

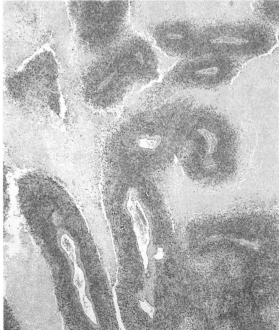

Fig. 3.12 Frontal meningioma. (F 74) Necrosis in this lesion has resulted in a papillary pattern although the cells are still clearly meningothelial. PS HE × 32

The psammomatous variant (Figs. 3.13 & 3.14) is marked by the presence of large numbers of psammoma bodies which develop from the deposition of calcium salts in the centre of the concentric cell whorls found in many meningiomas. These structures may also sometimes arise from vascular wall calcification and on occasions a meningioma may be almost entirely converted into a calcified mass (Fig. 3.15). Formation of psammoma bodies is often more marked in spinal than cranial meningiomas, but they are frequently found in smaller numbers in otherwise typical syncytial tumours.

In rare examples macroscopic calcification may be the result of metaplastic ossification within the connective tissue stroma of the tumour complete with the development of organised Haversian systems. Occasionally amyloid will be found deposited in vessel walls or fibrous stroma. Although striking, neither of these features have prognostic implications.

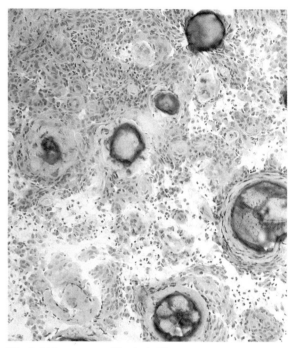

Fig. 3.14 Same case as Fig. 3.13. The structural relationship between cellular whorls and calcified psammoma bodies can be seen in this cryostat section. CS HE × 128

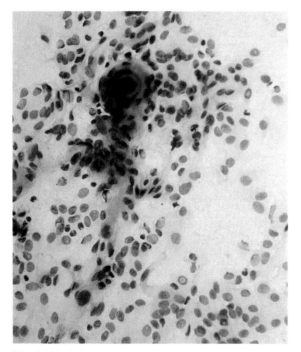

Fig. 3.13 Spinal meningioma. (F 57) Although calcified psammoma bodies may make smearing difficult the cells are still recognisably meningothelial. SP HE × 256

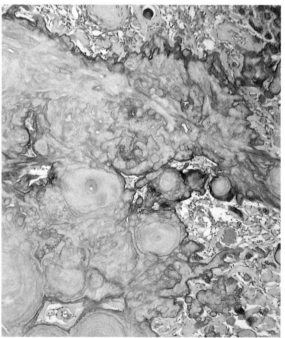

Fig. 3.15 Pineal region meningioma. (F 43) Massive confluent calcification has reduced the tumour tissue to an almost insignificant component (top). PS HE × 80

Fibroblastic meningiomas present a picture on cryostat sections (Fig. 3.16) of a spindle cell tumour, sometimes with an abundant collagenous stroma. Even in a tough fibrous tumour firm compression prior to smearing will usually expel cells which are diagnostic (Fig. 3.17). This may be of value in small biopsies which often show considerable surgical artefact on cryostat sections. The tumour cells are more flattened than spindle shaped and so, when cut in longitudinal section, appear fibroblastic but in tangential sections are more syncytial. In paraffin sections this may result in a pseudo-storiform pattern with a resemblance to fibrohistiocytic tumours (Fig. 3.18) that may be heightened by xanthoma cells. The combination of spindle cells and xanthoma cells may also resemble a neurilemoma (p. 82) although coarse collagen bands which are quite common in meningiomas, especially if fibroblastic, are rare in neurilemomas. Moreover the reticulin pattern of a meningioma is different (Fig. 3.12) and further distinction from a neurilemoma may be made by ultrastructural differences (p. 84) and the absence of S-100 protein staining.

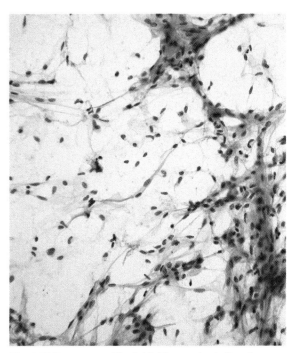

Fig. 3.17 Same case as Fig. 3.16. Elongated spindle cells are mixed with flattened, more typical meningothelial cells. SP HE × 205

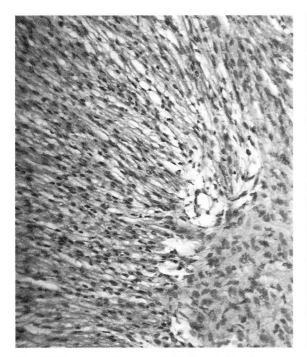

Fig. 3.16 Frontal meningioma. (F 67) The spindle cell appearances (left) which contrast with the syncytial zones depend partly on plane of section. CS HE × 205

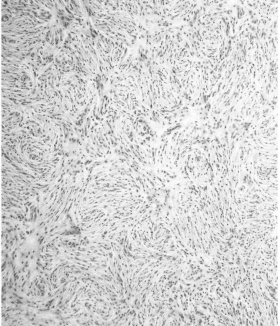

Fig. 3.18 Parietal meningioma. (F 36) A pseudo-storiform pattern results from the arrangement of spindle cells and syncytial areas. PS HE × 80

Myxomatous ground substance may be present in small amounts in many otherwise typical meningiomas. In the myxoid meningioma it is present in abundance and results in a sparsely cellular appearance on cryostat sections which is very different from a typical meningioma (Fig. 3.19). Smears (Fig. 3.20) will reveal the presence of cells with typical meningothelial features although they may be scarce and palely stained and careful searching of several preparations may be required.

In paraffin sections (Figs. 3.21 & 3.22) the true nature of the tumour is usually more obvious with foci of typical syncytial tumour although these may be scanty. The appearance of the tumour in paraffin sections is responsible for the alternative (but less accurate) term of microcystic meningioma. The myxoid matrix surrounding the tumour cells can be clearly seen in Alcian blue stained sections (Fig. 3.23) from regions of dural infiltration where acid glycosaminoglycans surround clusters of meningothelial cells.

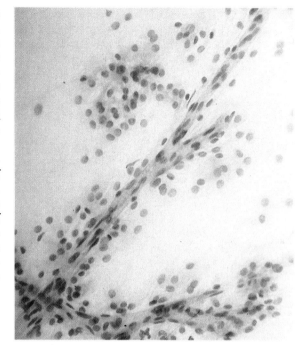

Fig. 3.20 Same case as Fig. 3.19. Although palely staining the regular cytology and pattern of clustering of tumour cells is more typically meningothelial. SP HE × 205

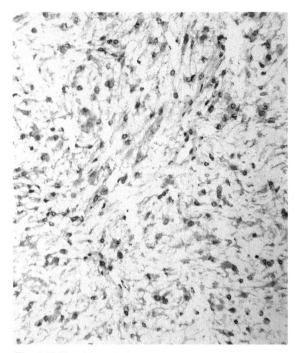

Fig. 3.19 Myxoid meningioma. (F 42) A meningeal nature is barely discernible due to the separation of fairly uniform cells by interstitial matrix. CS HE × 205

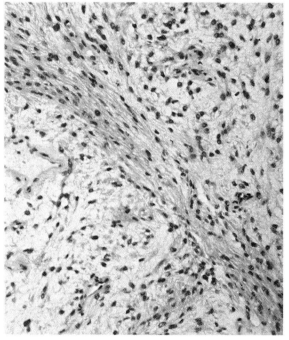

Fig. 3.21 Same case as Fig. 3.19. After paraffin processing the cells are more readily recognisable and some tumour architecture can be seen. PS HE × 205

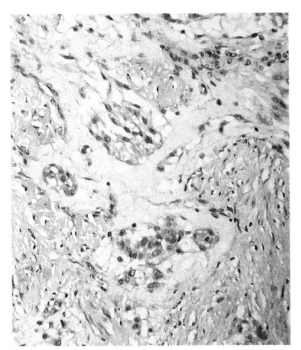

Fig. 3.22 Same case as Fig. 3.19. Small clusters of more obviously meningothelial cells lie within pools of basophilic matrix in infiltrated dura. PS HE × 205

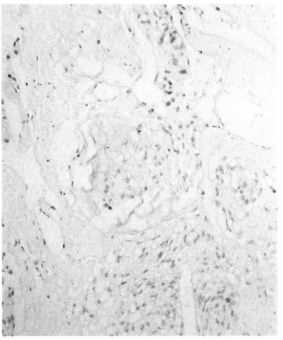

Fig. 3.23 Same case as Fig. 3.19. By appropriate staining the tumour matrix is shown to consist of acid glycosaminoglycans. PS AB × 205

ANGIOMATOUS MENINGIOMA

The angiomatous meningioma is a variant form in which the vascular elements of the stroma are prominent (Fig. 3.24), although the vessels are mature and not part of the neoplastic process. Difficulty may be encountered in distinguishing a small biopsy from a spinal tumour with this histology from a true angioma which not infrequently will have both intra-osseous and intra-dural portions. Careful searching may be necessary to identify scanty meningothelial elements, although these will usually have a typical whorled or syncytial arrangement. The term haemangioblastic has been applied to rare angiomatous meningiomas that are so vascular that they may be difficult to distinguish from capillary haemangioblastomas. These angiomatous tumours differ from other meningothelial lesions only in their vascularity and should not be confused with the haemangiopericytic meningioma (p. 66) which has an entirely different histology.

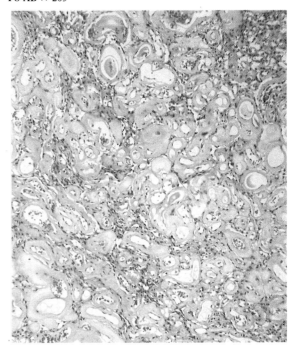

Fig. 3.24 Parasagittal meningioma. (F 63) Numerous blood vessels dominate the picture and compress residual tumour cells in this 'angiomatous' variant. PS HE × 80

The term atypical meningioma is applied to tumours which have a generally typical histology but in addition show three features that are not seen in the majority of meningiomas. These features are mitoses (Fig. 3.25), invasion of the cortex by tongues of tumour (Fig. 3.26) and multifocal necroses (Fig. 3.27) which should be contrasted with the central necrosis of large but otherwise typical tumours. Cortical invasion should be distinguished from simple indentation resulting from pressure atrophy which is quite common, especially in large meningiomas. Infiltration by single tumour cells is extremely rare.

This 'atypical' histology is commoner in tumours that have recurred and both cortical invasion and necrosis are commoner in tumours that subsequently recur, but there is no implication of overt malignancy with risk of metastasis. Although there is argument about the significance of these features, it does seem reasonable to recognise these lesions as differing histologically from other meningiomas to allow prospective correlation with other biological properties.

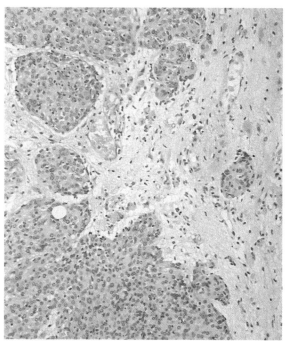

Fig. 3.26 Parietal atypical meningioma. (M 75) Multifocal invasion of cortex by tongues of tumour may predispose to local recurrence. PS HE × 128

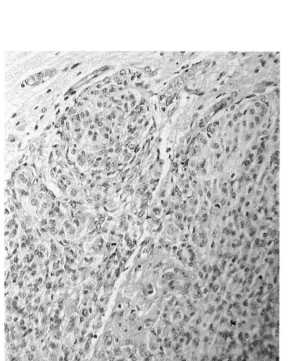

Fig. 3.25 Skull base atypical meningioma. (F 71) Cortical invasion (top) and the presence of mitoses are best assessed in paraffin sections. PS HE × 205

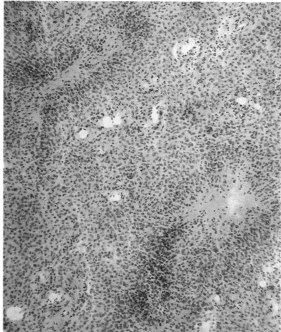

Fig. 3.27 Frontal atypical meningioma. (M 53) Multiple foci of necrosis in areas of otherwise typical histology are one feature of the 'atypical' tumour. CS HE × 80

FURTHER READING

Alguarcil-Garcia A, Pettigrew NM 1986 Secretory meningioma. A distinct subtype of meningioma. American Journal of Surgical Pathology 10:102–111

Borowich B, Doron Y 1986 Recurrence of intracranial meningiomas: the role played by regional multicentricity. Journal of Neurosurgery 64:58–63

Christensen D, Laursen H, Klinken L 1983 Prediction of recurrences in meningiomas after surgical treatment. A quantitative approach. Acta Neuropathologica (Berlin) 61:130–134

Crompton MR, Gautier-Smith PC 1970 The prediction of recurrence in meningiomas. Journal of Neurology Neurosurgery and Psychiatry 33:80–87

Jaaskelainen J, Haltia M, Servo A 1986 Atypical and anaplastic meningiomas: radiology, surgery, radiotherapy, and outcome. Surgical Neurology 25:233–242

Jellinger K, Slowik F 1975 Histological subtypes and prognostic problems in meningiomas. Journal of Neurology 208:279–298

Kepes JJ 1986 The histopathology of meningiomas. A reflection of origins and expected behavior? Journal of Neuropathology and Experimental Neurology 45:95–107

Marks SM, Whitwell HL, Lye RH 1986 Recurrence of meningiomas after operation. Surgical Neurology 25:436–440

Meis JM, Ordonez NG, Bruner JM 1986 Meningiomas: an immunohistochemical study of 50 cases. Archives of Pathology and Laboratory Medicine 110:934–937

Michaud J, Gagne F 1983 Microcystic meningioma. Clinicopathologic report of eight cases. Archives of Pathology and Laboratory Medicine 107:75–80

de la Monte SM, Flickinger J, Linggood RM 1986 Histopathologic features predicting recurrence of meningiomas following subtotal resection. American Journal of Surgical Pathology 10:836–843

Pasquier B, Gasnier F, Pasquier D, Keddari E, Morens A, Couderc P 1986 Papillary meningioma: clinicopathologic study of seven cases and review of the literature. Cancer 58: 299–305

Schnitt SJ, Vogel H 1986 Meningiomas. Diagnostic value of immunoperoxidase staining for epithelial membrane antigen. American Journal of Surgical Pathology 10:640–649

Skullerud K, Loken AC 1974 The prognosis in meningiomas. Acta Neuropathologica (Berlin) 29:337–344

Theaker JM, Gatter KC, Esiri MM, Fleming KA 1986 Epithelial membrane antigen and cytokeratin expression by meningiomas: an immunohistological study. Journal of Clinical Pathology 39:435–439

NOTES

This meningeal tumour differs from meningothelial lesions both in its histology and, more importantly, its behaviour. It most probably arises from the perivascular cell (pericyte) of the meningeal vessels and as such is allied in nature to haemangiopericytomas arising in other locations. Although usually entirely of this type lesions do occur in which both haemangiopericytic and typical meningothelial areas are found. Whether these represent mixed tumours or provide evidence for a meningothelial origin for the haemangiopericytic meningioma is not clear. This controversy is in part reflected in the use of the alternative name of angioblastic meningioma for these tumours. The importance of distinguishing this tumour from meningothelial meningiomas lies in its increased risk of recurrence and its generally more aggressive behaviour.

In cryostat sections (Fig. 3.28) the higher cellularity is immediately apparent as is the number of small vessels, often compressed but discernible on close examination. The tumour cells have great cohesion due to their intercellular external laminae and smears differ radically from those of meningothelial tumours. Few single cells separate from smeared fragments (Fig. 3.29), but where they can be visualised they are generally smaller than meningothelial cells with little cytoplasm. Mitoses may be readily apparent but this is not inevitable. The vasculocentric arrangement of the cells is usually obvious in paraffin sections (Fig. 3.30), and while some rudimentary whorling may be seen this is perivascular and not an indication of a meningothelial nature. In larger specimens areas of necrosis, fibrosis (Fig. 3.31) or extensive stromal hyalinization are common. In some lesions the vasculocentric pattern may not be so clear and cells may occur in sheets (Fig. 3.32), sometimes within a hyaline matrix. Any doubts about the lesion's nature will be resolved by examination of a reticulin stain (Fig. 3.33) which emphasises the vascular pattern and demonstrates the non-meningothelial pattern of the pericellular basement membrane that is typical of the haemangiopericytic meningioma.

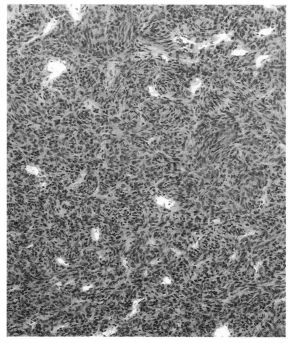

Fig. 3.28 Occipital haemangiopericytic meningioma. (F 34) The high cellularity and numerous compressed vessels are easy to appreciate in a cryostat section. CS HE × 128

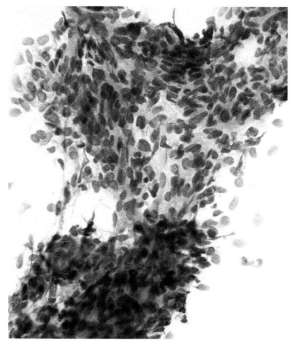

Fig. 3.29 Same case as Fig. 3.28. The cohesive nature of the tumour tissue rather than its cytology distinguishes it from meningothelial lesions. SP HE × 320

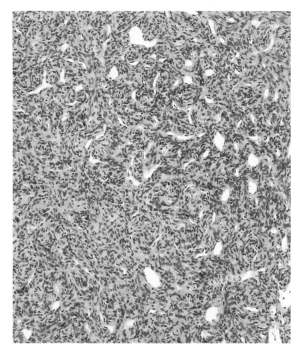

Fig. 3.30 Same tissue as Fig. 3.28. After paraffin processing the number of blood vessels and the vasculocentric arrangement of cells is easier to discern. CP HE × 128

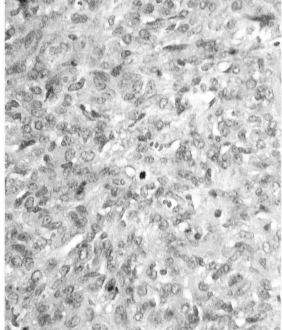

Fig. 3.32 Same case as Fig. 3.31. A perivascular pattern is not universal but the tumour cells lack the uniformity of meningothelial lesions. PS HE × 320

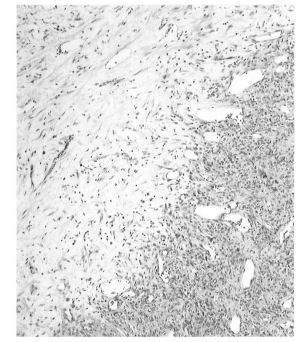

Fig. 3.31 Parasagittal haemangiopericytic meningioma. (F 48) Cellular tissue borders on a zone of fibrosis (top) that has resulted from tumour necrosis. PS HE × 80

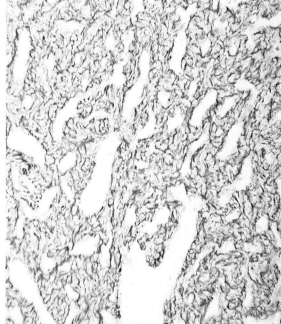

Fig. 3.33 Same case as Fig. 3.28. The vascular pattern and the extent of pericellular basement membrane contrasts with a typical meningothelial tumour. PS RETIC × 205

Malignant tumours of meningeal origin are usually primary sarcomas, but malignant change (and sometimes sarcoma development) may occur in pre-existing meningiomas. Rare primary malignant melanomas also develop from the melanocytes that are normally present in the meninges. The sarcomas that are encountered are usually fibrosarcomas or, less commonly, angiosarcomas arising from the connective tissue of the meninges or their vessels. Malignant fibrous histiocytomas are increasingly being recognised in this location although fibroblastic meningiomas may mimic fibrohistiocytic tumours (Fig. 3.18). Rare chondrosarcomas and osteosarcomas have also been described. Histologically they show the features that would be expected in such lesions occurring in other sites. Fibrosarcomas demonstrate unequivocal histological features of malignancy on cryostat sections (Fig. 3.34), and smear appearances indicating a cohesive spindle cell tumour (Fig. 3.35). Exact classification of meningeal sarcomas is usually better done using paraffin sections (Fig. 3.36) when many areas can be sampled and studied.

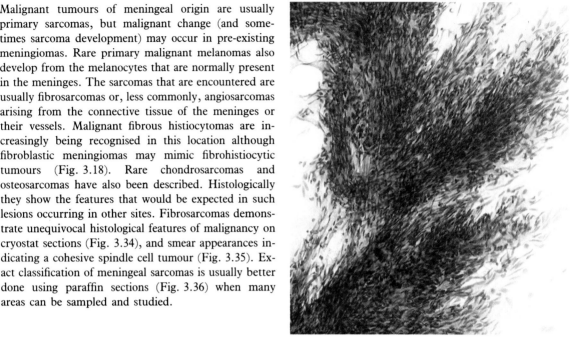

Fig. 3.35 Same case as Fig. 3.34. The cell density, cytology and cohesion of the component spindle cells can be appreciated on this smear. SP HE × 160

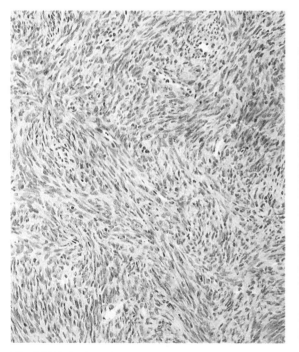

Fig. 3.34 Parietal meningeal sarcoma. (M 43) The high cellularity and fascicular pattern of a fibrosarcoma distinguishes this particular example. CS HE × 256

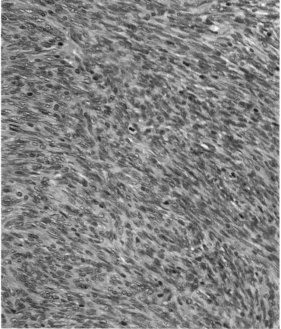

Fig. 3.36 Same case as Fig. 3.34. Paraffin sections show the typical appearances of a fibrosarcoma. PS HE × 320

FURTHER READING

Cybulski GR, Russell EJ, D'Angelo CM, Bailey OT 1985
Falcine chondrosarcoma: case report and literature review.
Neurosurgery 16:412–415

Holden J, Dolman CL, Churg A 1987 Immunohistochemistry
of meningiomas including the angioblastic type. Journal of
Neuropathology and Experimental Neurology 46:50–56

Horten BC, Urich H, Rubinstein LJ, Montague SR 1977 The
angioblastic meningioma: a reappraisal of a nosological
problem. Journal of the Neurological Sciences 31:387–410

Lam RNY, Malik GM, Chason JL 1981 Osteosarcoma of
meninges. Clinical, light, and ultrastructural observations of
a case. American Journal of Surgical Pathology 5:302–208

Nakamura M, Inoue HK, Ono N, Kunimune H, Tamada J
1987 Analysis of hemangiopericytic meningiomas by
immunohistochemistry, electron microscopy and cell
culture. Journal of Neuropathology and Experimental
Neurology 46:57–71

Schrantz JL, Araoz CA 1972 Radiation induced meningeal
fibrosarcoma. Archives of Pathology and Laboratory
Medicine 93:26–31

Silber SW, Smith KR, Horenstein S 1978 Primary
leptomeningeal melanoma. An ultrastructural study. Cancer
41:519–527

Swamy KSN, Shankar SK, Asha T, Reddy AK 1986
Malignant fibrous histiocytoma arising from the meninges of
the posterior fossa. Surgical Neurology 25:18–24

Pena CE 1975 Intracranial hemangiopericytoma.
Ultrastructural evidence of its leiomyoblastic differentiation.
Acta Neuropathologica (Berlin) 33:279–284

Weiss SW, Enzinger FM 1978 Malignant fibrous histiocytoma:
analysis of 200 cases. Cancer 41:2250–2267

NOTES

4 PRIMITIVE NEUROECTODERMAL AND NEURONAL TUMOURS

The use of the term primitive neuroectodermal tumour (PNET) has been advocated for a group of tumours that, although rare, are more common in childhood and have features that suggest that they are derived from a primitive glial or neuronal precursor cell with a potential for multiple differentiation. This approach has the practical advantage of recognising a basic similarity among a group of lesions that may show considerable histological diversity but similar clinical behaviour.

Primitive neuroectodermal tumours are currently classified on the basis of their demonstrable differentiation and increasing use is being made of immunohistochemical techniques to refine this process. The primitive cells that compose the tumour may form characteristic rosettes with central fibrillary zones consisting of cell processes (Fig. 4.1) although it is often difficult to prove that the cells forming these structures are demonstrating any specific differentiation. Astrocytic differentiation may be suggested on routine sections but demonstration of GFAP expression is usually necessary for confirmation. In the rosettes described above, or in areas devoid of specific architecture, neuroblastic differentiation may be demonstrated with markers such as 'neurone specific' enolase or neurofilament protein, or by ultrastructural identification of neurosecretory granules. Neuronal differentiation with ganglion cell development is rare and may be difficult of distinguish from residual non-neoplastic neurones. Ependymal differentiation will be evident as ependymal tubules (Fig. 2.94), and in the absence of a consistent marker of neoplastic oligodendrocytes identification of oligodendroglial differentiation relies on the histological feature of regular perinuclear haloes (Fig. 4.2). The significance of tumour differentiation seems to vary with site but is associated with a poorer outcome in cerebellar lesions and a better one in the cerebrum. Many of these tumours show multiple differentiation supporting the view that they should be considered as a family rather than as separate primitive tumour classes, although this is not universally accepted.

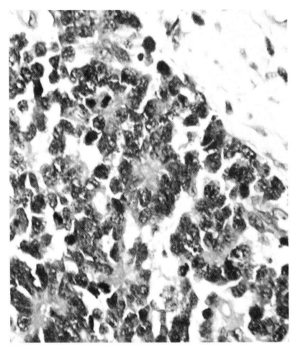

Fig. 4.1 Cerebral PNET. (M 6 months) The fibrillary centre of these rosettes contrasts with the lumen of ependymoblastic tubules (Fig. 2.94). PS HE × 512

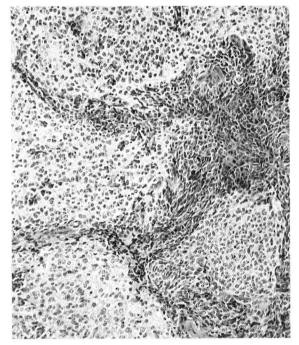

Fig. 4.2 Cerebellar PNET. (F 4) Areas of oligodendroglial cells with well defined perinuclear haloes contrast with primitive areas of higher cellularity PS HE × 128

PNETs occur most commonly in the cerebellum and for many years the synonym of medulloblastoma has been used. The lesions may be situated in the midline or laterally within a hemisphere, the former being the commoner site in younger children.

In smears (Fig. 4.3) and cryostat sections (Fig. 4.4) the primitive nature of the cells is readily apparent, with sheets of undifferentiated cells with hyperchromatic nuclei, often abundant mitoses and scanty process formation. In smears from the cerebellum great care must be exercised if a piece of normal granular layer is not to be misinterpreted as tumour although the granular cell neurones are generally smaller than most tumour cells (Fig. 4.3). The presence of a regular zone of Purkinje cells, a clear border with adjacent white matter and the intermixed population of supporting glia distinguish normal granular layer from tumour. The neuroglial nature of PNETs will usually be apparent at the infiltrating edge where perineuronal and perivascular secondary structures may be seen (Fig. 4.5).

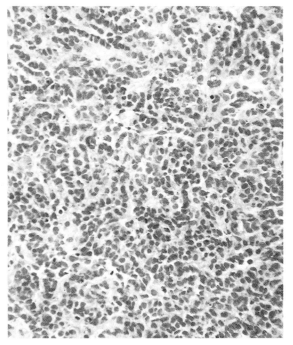

Fig. 4.4 Cerebellar PNET. (F 18) Few specific architectural features can be discerned in cryostat sections from most cerebellar PNETs. CS HE × 256

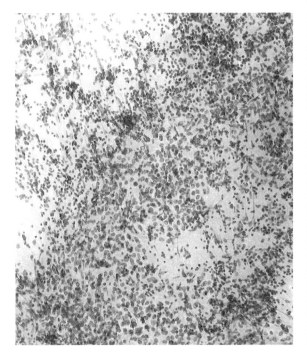

Fig. 4.3 Cerebellar PNET. (M 36) Primitive tumour cells (centre) contrast with the smaller neurones of the granular layer (top left). SP HE × 128

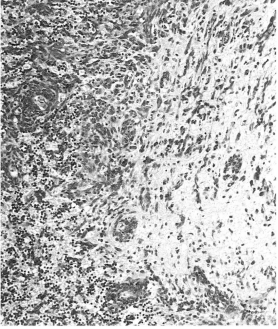

Fig. 4.5 Cerebellar PNET. (M 22) At the junction of tumour with cerebellum (right) a pattern of perivascular and single cell infiltration is seen. PS HE × 128

Tumour cells frequently infiltrate into the meninges and metastasise via the CSF (Fig. 4.6). On occasions a marked mesenchymal response may be evoked which may result in a distortion of the tumour architecture by collagen (Fig. 4.7) or actively proliferating mesenchymal cells which may resemble a sarcoma. This 'desmoplastic' variant is characterised by abundant reticulin (Fig. 4.8) (derived from mesenchymal rather than tumour cells) and is associated with a more favourable prognosis than more typical tumours, possibly because the greater demarcation that results aids excision. A tumour may occasionally cause confusion by presenting as a cerebellopontine lesion due to direct infiltration into cranial nerves.

A PNET may resemble lymphoma (Fig. 6.2) or metastatic small cell carcinoma (Fig. 14.7) and the site of the lesion, the age of the patient and the clinical history should all be taken into account before reaching a diagnosis. PNET cells tend to separate less than lymphomas, do not form the discrete clumps seen in carcinomas and the tumours rarely show extensive necrosis.

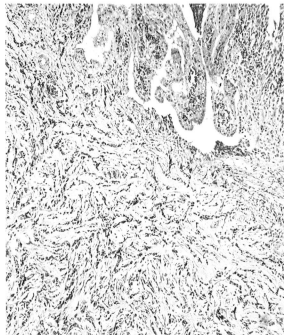

Fig. 4.7 Cerebellar PNET. (F 4) Infiltration of choroid and leptomeninges is associated with collagen production that distorts and compresses tumour cells. PS HE × 80

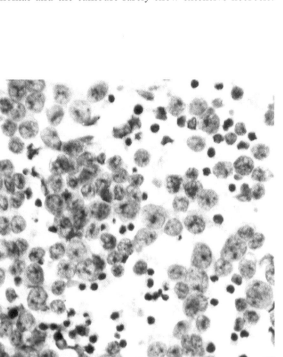

Fig. 4.6 Cerebellar PNET. (F 3) Tumour cells in the CSF were associated with deposits in the lumbar subarachnoid space. CYTO GIEM × 512

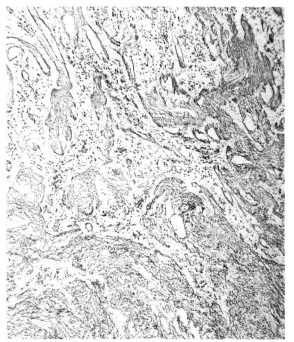

Fig. 4.8 Same case as Fig. 4.7. The perivascular origin of much of the connective tissue in a 'desmoplastic' response is emphasised by a reticulin stain. PS RETIC × 80

This is a rare tumour, occurring in children or young adults, with histological features (Figs. 4.9–4.11) similar to such lesions of the cerebellum although there may be greater diversity in differentiation in a larger proportion of cases. It is said to be more resistant to treatment. Tumours in which primitive cells form structures similar to embryonic neural tube (Fig. 4.10) have been termed medulloepitheliomas although the presence of ependymal features in some (Fig. 4.11) casts doubt on the validity of this distinction.

Cerebral PNETs should be distinguished from occasional glioblastomas in which areas with a 'small cell' pattern may be seen. In these the primary tumour structure is that of a glioblastoma in which primitive areas are present, which contrasts with a PNET which is composed predominantly of primitive cells some of which may show specific differentiation.

Occasionally tumours are encountered (usually in children) with a mixture of PNET and oligodendroglioma or astrocytoma in which discrete areas of two distinct tumour types co-exist.

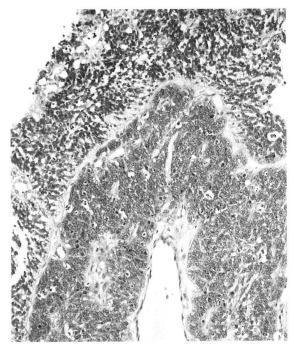

Fig. 4.10 Same case as Fig. 4.9. 'Epithelial' areas which resemble the cells of primitive neural tube are seen intermixed with smaller primitive cells. PS HE × 128

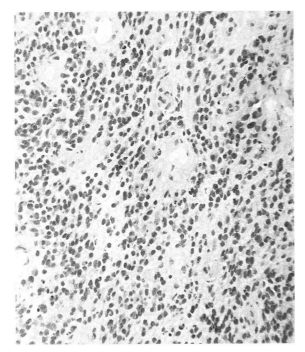

Fig. 4.9 Cerebral PNET. (F 4) Perivascular orientation in places suggests an ependymoma but mitoses and meningeal invasion were also present. CS HE × 205

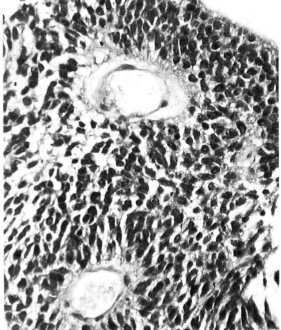

Fig. 4.11 Same tissue as Fig. 4.9. The primitive nature of the cells and a focal perivascular pattern are evident in paraffin processed tissue. CP HE × 320

Central neuroblastomas are rare and are best considered as PNETs showing solely neuroblastic differentiation (p. 72).

Also rare, the ganglioglioma is a lesion most commonly occurring in the region of the third ventricle in the young, in which mature but abnormal, ganglion cells are mixed with varying amounts of glial and mesenchymal tissue. Where the glial elements predominate areas indistinguishable from an astrocytoma will be seen. The admixture of cells may be diffuse (Fig. 4.12 & 4.13) or clusters of ganglion cells may be enclosed by non-neuronal elements which often form abundant reticulin (Fig. 4.14). Examples composed entirely of neuronal and axonal elements without a glial component are termed ganglioneuromas but this distinction is rarely clear. On rare occasions the glial component may undergo malignant change or a PNET may develop in a pre-existing ganglioglioma. Occasional examples are encountered in which a ganglioglioma develops from a PNET suggesting that some lesions may develop from primitive neuroblastic precursors in a manner homologous to the peripheral ganglioneuroblastoma.

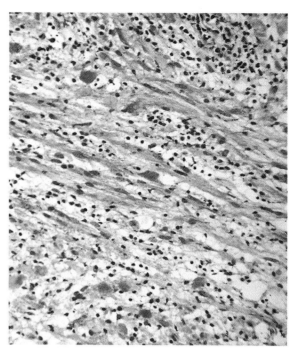

Fig. 4.13 Same case as Fig. 4.12. Ganglion cells are intermixed with glial elements and a lymphoid infiltrate which is not uncommon in these lesions. CS HE × 80

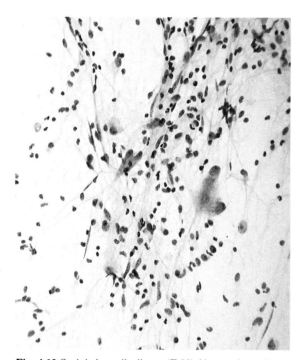

Fig. 4.12 Occipital ganglioglioma. (F 22) Abnormal ganglion cells, some binucleate, are mixed with spindle shaped glial cells. SP HE × 205

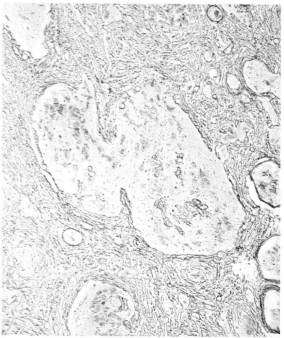

Fig. 4.14 Cerebellar ganglioglioma. (F 2) The predominantly neuronal areas are enclosed by a mixture of glial cells and reticulin-forming elements. PS RETIC × 80

FURTHER READING

Beale MF, Kleinman GM, Ojeman RG, Hochberg FH 1981 Gangliocytoma of the third ventricle : hyperphagia, somnolence and dementia. Neurology 31:1224–1228

Burger PC, Grahmann FC, Bliestle A, Kleihues P 1987 Differentiation in the medulloblastoma. A histological and immunohistochemical study. Acta Neuropathologica (Berlin) 73:115–123

Caputy AJ, McCullough DC, Manz HJ, Patterson K, Hammock MK 1987 A review of factors influencing the prognosis of medulloblastoma. The importance of differentiation. Journal of Neurosurgery 66:80–87

de Chadarevian J-P, Montes JL, O'Gorman A, Freeman CR 1987 Maturation of cerebellar neuroblastoma into ganglioneuroma with melanosis. Cancer 59:69–76

Chatty EM, Earle KM 1971 Medulloblastoma. A report of 201 cases with emphasis on the relationship of histologic variants to survival. Cancer 28:977–983

Dastur DK 1982 Cerebral ganglioglio-neuroblastoma : an unusual brain tumour of the neuron series. Journal of Neurology Neurosurgery and Psychiatry 45:139–142

Dehner LP 1986 Peripheral and central primitive neuroectodermal tumours. A nosologic concept seeking a consensus. Archives of Pathology and Laboratory Medicine 110:997–1005

Gaffney CC, Sloane JP, Bradley NJ, Bloom HJG 1985 Primitive neuroectodermal tumours of the cerebrum. Journal of Neuro-Oncology 3:23–33

Johannsson JH, Rekate HL, Roessmann U 1981 Gangliogliomas: pathological and clinical correlation. Journal of Neurosurgery 54:58–63

MacKenzie JMM, Franks AJ, van Hille PT, Cameron MM 1987 The evolution of an oligodendroglioma into a primitive neuroectodermal tumour. Neuropathology and Applied Neurobiology 13:in press.

Pearl GS, Takei Y 1981 Cerebellar 'neuroblastoma': nosology as it relates to medulloblastoma. Cancer 47:772–779

Packer RJ, Sutton LN, Rorke LB, Littman PA, Sposto R, Rosenstock JG, Bruce DA, Schut L 1984 Prognostic importance of cellular differentiation in medulloblastoma of childhood. Journal of Neurosurgery 61:296–301

Rhodes RH, Davis RL, Kassel SH, Clague BH 1978 Primary cerebral neuroblastoma: a light and electron microscopic study. Acta Neuropathologica (Berl) 41:119–124

Rorke LB 1983 The cerebellar medulloblastoma and its relationship to primitive neuroectodermal tumors. Journal of Neuropathology and Experimental Neurology 42:1–15

Rorke LB, Gilles FH, Davis RL, Becker LE 1985 Revision of the World Health Organisation classification of brain tumors for childhood brain tumors. Cancer 56:1869–1886

Rubinstein LJ 1985 A commentary on the proposed revision of the World Health Organisation classification of brain tumors for childhood brain tumors. Cancer 56:1887–1888

Rubinstein LJ 1985 Embryonal central neuroepithelial tumors and their differentiating potential. A cytogenetic view of a complex neuro-oncological problem. Journal of Neurosurgery 62:795–805

Sato T, Shimoda A, Takahashi T, Daita G, Goto S, Takamura H, Hirama M 1980 Congenital cerebellar neuroepithelial tumor with multiple divergent differentiations. Acta Neuropathologica (Berl) 50:143–146

Sawa H, Takeshita I, Kuramitsu M, Mannoji H, Machi T, Fukui M, Kitamura K 1986 Neuronal and glial proteins in medulloblastomas I Immunohistochemical studies. Anticancer Research 6:905–910.

Tang TT, Harb JM, Mork SJ, Sty JR 1985 Composite cerebral neuroblastoma and astrocytoma. Cancer 56:1404–1412

NOTES

5 NERVE SHEATH TUMOURS

This tumour is derived from Schwann cells (hence its alternative name of Schwannoma) of the cranial nerves and spinal nerve roots. It develops distal to the sites of nerve emergence from the brain stem or spinal cord, at or beyond the point of changeover from central oligodendroglial myelination to peripheral myelination by Schwann cells. The tumours are mostly found on sensory nerves and only rarely involve purely motor nerves. The intracranial variety is most commonly located on the vestibular branch of the eighth nerve (acoustic neuroma) whilst the intraspinal variety usually grows on dorsal roots. Multiple tumours do occur but are particularly associated with bilateral acoustic (central) neurofibromatosis, and practically all cases of bilateral eighth nerve neurilemomas occur in the context of this condition. Cases in which a typical histology is associated with melanin production emphasise the common origin of Schwann cells and melanocytes. Further consideration is given to pigmented nerve sheath tumours on page 88.

The tumour grows by expansion beneath the perineurial sheath and so is contained within a connective tissue 'capsule', compressing the nerve of origin which is peripherally displaced (Fig. 5.1). As a result axons are not found within the tissue that makes up the tumour except at the edges where it merges with the nerve. This contrasts with the situation in a neurofibroma (p. 87) where axons form an integral part of the lesion.

The constituent cells are surrounded to a greater or lesser extent by an external lamina which gives great cohesion but variations in the amount of interstitial matrix and fluid result in two major tissue patterns. Designated Antoni A and B they correspond respectively to areas of compact spindle cells and areas in which cells of variable morphology are separated by a prominent interstitial matrix. Haemorrhage, lipid-laden cells and lymphocytic infiltration are also features found in Antoni B tissue. These two patterns are best recognised in sections but their physical characteristics determine their appearances in smears.

Irrespective of Antoni type the presence of an external lamina is responsible for the way in which the tumour smears. Single cells do not separate and the smeared specimen fragments into pieces which remain cohesive (Fig. 5.2). This feature is most obvious in Antoni A tissue and cell detail may be difficult to discern, but at the edges the cytology of the component spindle cells is normally visible (Fig. 5.2). Areas of lower cell density correspond to Antoni B tissue (Fig. 5.3), with interstitial matrix separating the cells into strands. Within these the cells are far less regular and considerable pleomorphism may be seen (Fig. 5.4). Where separated cells are seen in any number they are usually lymphocytes or lipid-laden cells rather than neoplastic cells and can be seen to differ from the cells that make up the larger fragments. Recognition of the coherent nature of the smeared fragments is of far more diagnostic value than the specific identification of Antoni A and B tissue which are simply ends of a structural spectrum, a fact that is reinforced when junctional zones between the two are studied (Figs. 5.5 & 5.6).

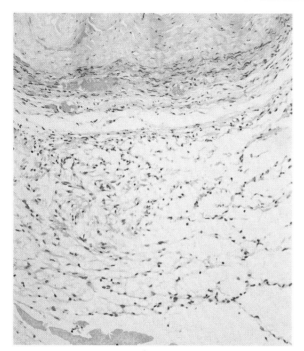

Fig. 5.1 Spinal neurilemoma. (F 33) Tumour (below) compresses remnants of the nerve from which it has arisen against the perineurium (above). PS HE × 128

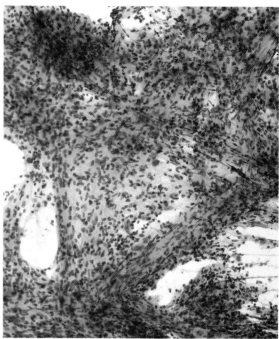

Fig. 5.3 Eighth nerve neurilemoma. (F 64) In Antoni B tissue the cells are more variable, and both haemorrhage and a lymphocytic infiltrate may be seen. SP HE × 128

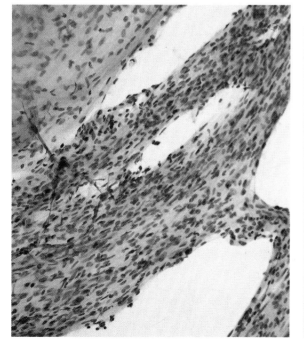

Fig. 5.2 Eighth nerve neurilemoma. (F 55) The spindle form of the cells in Antoni A tissue and the clear margins of the tumour fragments can be seen. SP HE × 205

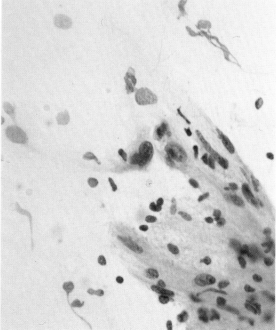

Fig. 5.4 Same case as Fig. 5.3. At higher magnification the degree of pleomorphism may be alarming, although the lack of cell separation is obvious. SP HE × 400

In cryostat sections (Figs. 5.5. & 5.6) the distinction between the two tumour patterns is not always obvious and there may be more than a superficial resemblance to an astrocytoma. The coherent non-glial appearances of the smear should lead to realisation that the 'loose' appearances are due to extracellular matrix (which may be metachromatic on toluidine blue stained cryostat sections) rather than interstitial fluid (as is generally the case in an astrocytoma). Malignancy may be considered because of the cellular pleomorphism which is a frequent finding in Antoni B areas, but appreciation that mitoses are absent in areas of cellular atypia will prevent such an error.

Paraffin sections (Fig. 5.7) show the dimorphic picture of compact spindle cells comprising Antoni A tissue, and more loosely textured areas comprising type B tissue. The spindle cells in Antoni A areas may be arranged in a characteristic pattern with nuclear alignment resulting in a palisaded appearance (Fig. 5.8) and occasionally lamellated structures resembling peripheral sensory receptors may develop (Verocay bodies), but these, and well developed palisading, are both commoner in spinal than cranial neurilemomas.

Blood vessels in the neurilemoma often have a surrounding cuff of hyaline collagen (Figs. 5.6 & 5.7) although the poorer support provided by Antoni B tissue is probably responsible for the frequency with which haemorrhage (both old and recent) and vascular thrombosis are found in these lesions. A patchy infiltrate of lymphocytes is common and lipid-laden cells (Fig. 5.9) are also a frequent finding. Small cysts may also be found in Antoni B areas and occasionally the lesion may be largely cystic leading to an operative diagnosis of dermoid or epidermoid cyst, or even of astrocytoma.

Such cystic change is often more obvious in cases which have an unusual degree of stromal collagenisation (Fig. 5.10) which results in large hyaline areas with scattered aggregates of foam cells, and areas of spindle cells. These lesions have been described as 'ancient' neurilemomas but the appearances may not truly represent ageing changes so much as the effects of chronic ischaemia.

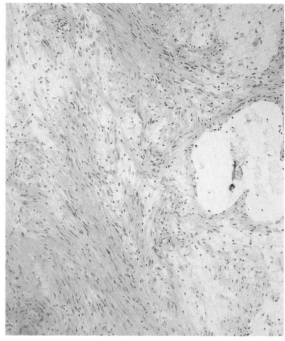

Fig. 5.5 Eighth nerve neurilemoma. (F 55) There is a contrast between the compact Antoni A and looser Antoni B tissue although transition is obvious. CS HE× 80

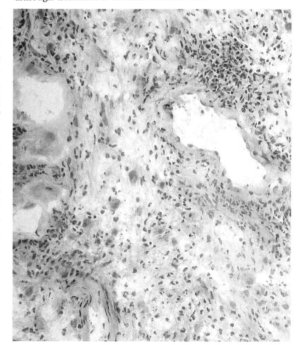

Fig. 5.6 Eighth nerve neurilemoma. (F 64) Antoni B tissue shows cellular variation, lymphocytic infiltration and collagenous perivascular 'collars'. CS HE × 160

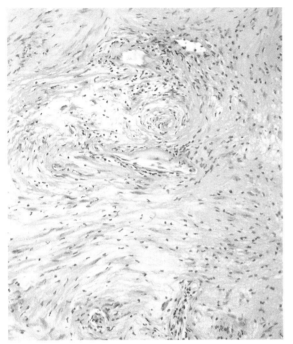

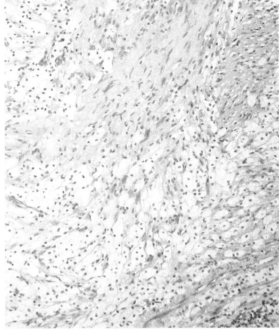

Fig. 5.7 Same case as Fig. 5.5. After paraffin processing there is a greater contrast between the two tissue types but similarities remain. CP HE × 128

Fig. 5.9 Eighth nerve neurilemoma. (F 67) Lipid laden cells separate spindle cells in an area transitional between Antoni A and B. PS HE × 128

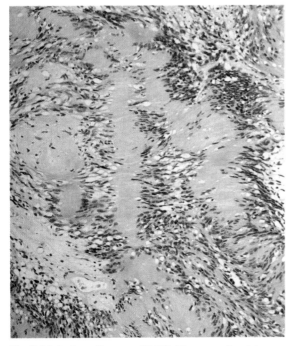

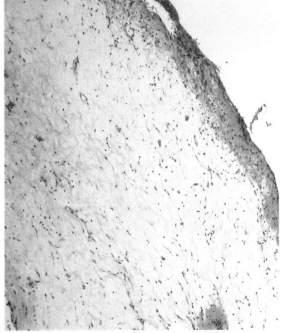

Fig. 5.8 Spinal neurilemoma. (M 39) Alignment of nuclei results in palisading in Antoni A tissue although it is not always as obvious as this. PS HE × 128

Fig. 5.10 Fifth nerve neurilemoma. (F 52) Only small areas of recognisable spindle cell tumour remain in the wall of a largely cystic lesion. PS HE × 80

Where a biopsy consists entirely of Antoni type A tissue distinction from a fibroblastic meningioma (p. 61) may be difficult. A smear should provide most help in distinguishing the two lesions, but in the absence of unfixed tissue the reticulin pattern and staining for S-100 protein will be of value.

In neurilemomas (Fig. 5.11) the reticulin is finely, though widely, distributed (reflecting the presence of pericellular external lamina) but usually without the development of large amounts of intercellular collagen. This contrasts with the reticulin pattern in a meningioma which is far coarser and more irregular with areas devoid of reticulin usually being found (Fig. 3.6).

When collagen is present in a neurilemoma it is usually fine and regular (Fig. 5.12), both between cells and around vessels. Collagen in a meningioma, however, is usually coarse and in thicker bundles, and may consist in part of invaded dura rather than entirely tumour-derived collagen. Calcification is extremely rare in neurilemomas, and if present (especially in the form of calcospherites) in a predominantly spindle cell tumour would suggest that the lesion is a meningioma rather than a neurilemoma.

Immunohistochemically S-100 protein is present in the majority of neurilemomas. Reaction is seen in cells of both Antoni A and Antoni B tissues with staining of nuclei or cytoplasm or both (Fig. 5.13). In contrast meningiomas only rarely show staining with polyclonal antisera and even then the nuclear staining is never as intense. Ultrastructurally the characteristic features of the tumour (Figs. 5.14 & 5.15) are numerous interdigitating cell processes frequently with surrounding external lamina, peripheral membrane densities, nondesmosomal cell junctions, finely dispersed intermediate filaments, occasional lipid droplets and small numbers of normal intracellular organelles. These appearances contrast sufficiently with those of a meningioma (which has abundant desmosomal junctions, often dense intermediate filaments and no external lamina) (Fig. 3.5) to be of value in distinguishing the two.

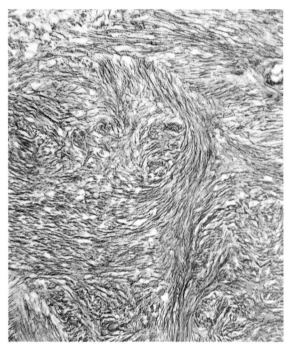

Fig. 5.11 Eighth nerve neurilemoma. (M 49) The reticulin is uniformly distributed around individual cells with no areas devoid of staining. PS RETIC × 205

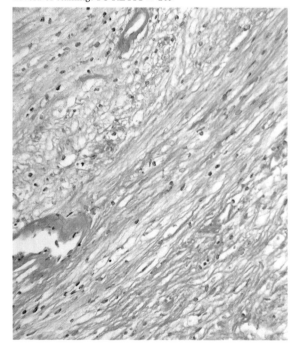

Fig. 5.12 Same case as Fig. 5.11. Collagen is present around blood vessels and as fine fibres between cells but does not form coarse bundles. PS VAN G × 205

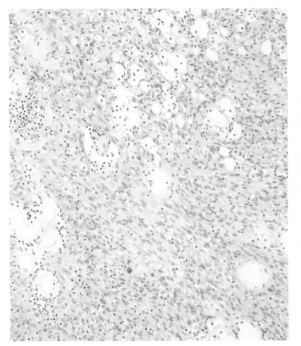

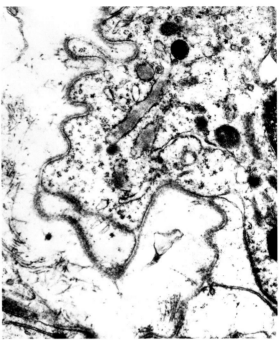

Fig. 5.13 Fifth nerve neurilemoma. (F 52) S-100 protein is present in most cells in tissue of Antoni A (below) and B (above) type. PS IP S-100 × 128

Fig. 5.15 Same case as Fig. 5.14. At higher magnification the pericellular external lamina is clearer as are the intracytoplasmic contents. EM × 19 380

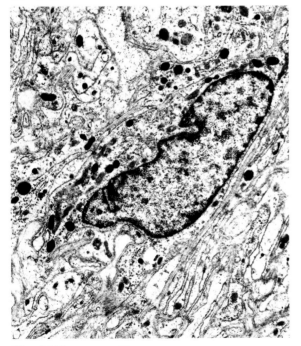

Fig. 5.14 Same case as Fig. 5.13. Interdigitating cell processes surround a single cell body, with some discernible intervening external lamina. EM × 4785

FURTHER READING

Dahl I 1977 Ancient neurilemmoma (Schwannoma). Acta
    Pathologica Microbiologica et Immunologica Scandinavica
    Sect. A 85:812–818
Dahl I, Hagmar B, Idvall I 1984 Benign solitary neurilemoma
    (schwannoma)—a correlative cytological and histological
    study of 28 cases. Acta Pathologica Microbiologica et
    Immunologica Scandinavica Sect. A 92:91–101

Miller RT, Sarikaya H, Sos A 1986 Melanotic schwannoma of
    the acoustic nerve. Archives of Pathology and Laboratory
    Medicine 110:153–154
Sobel RA, Michaud J 1985 Microcystic meningioma of the falx
    cerebri with numerous palisaded structures: an unusual
    histological pattern mimicking schwannoma. Acta
    Neuropathologica (Berlin) 68:256–258

NOTES

This tumour-like lesion is characteristic of Von Recklinghausen's (peripheral) neurofibromatosis. It is composed of all the constituents of the normal nerve (Schwann cells, fibroblasts, axons and mast cells) and may be found wherever peripheral myelinated nerves occur. In relation to the central nervous system it most commonly involves the spinal nerve roots, either within the dural sheath or, more commonly, by extension from a lesion in the retropleural or retroperitoneal space. Although probably a hamartoma rather than a neoplasm it shows progressive growth, has a definite risk of recurrence after excision, and is the lesion in which many neurofibrosarcomas develop. For this reason, if for no other, distinction from a neurilemoma is important and should be made.

Two main patterns are seen: plexiform, in which the nerve trunks are diffusely enlarged but remain discrete; and diffuse, in which some elements of the lesion extend beyond the confines of the nerve sheath into the adjacent tissues. These distinctions are not always clear and probably of little prognostic import.

On cryostat sections (Fig. 5.16) the lesion has a loose appearance with haphazardly arranged spindle cells forming an irregularly 'wavy' pattern, sometimes aligned with, or enclosing fine bands of collagen. Axons are usually found within the tumour substance and their presence within the lesion is a useful distinguishing feature from a neurilemoma. The high proportion of collagen and matrix to cells renders neurofibromas virtually impossible to smear.

Paraffin sections (Fig. 5.17) reveal the typical structure and may also show the presence of scattered atypical cells that are without significance in terms of predicting growth rate, risk of recurrence or malignant change. Where there is a history of recent rapid enlargement multiple samples should be examined to exclude the possibility that a sarcoma has developed.

Individuals with neurofibromatosis are liable to develop a wide range of nervous system tumours. As a result biopsies from such patients are as likely to be from meningiomas, astrocytomas, or neurilemomas, as they are to be from neurofibromas.

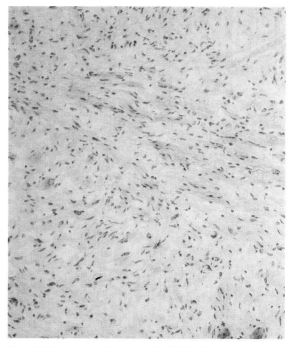

Fig. 5.16 Spinal neurofibroma. (M 27) Myelinated axons (running horizontally at top) can be seen within the lesion. CS HE × 128

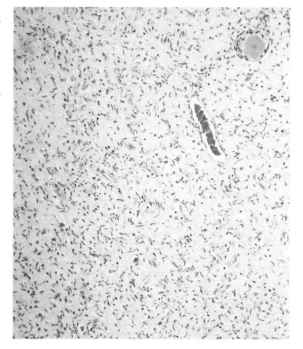

Fig. 5.17 Same case as Fig. 5.16. The components of this lesion (which involves a dorsal root ganglion) are easier to see after paraffin processing. PS HE × 128

The first category includes tumours which arise from a nerve, are histologically malignant and have features of a recognisable nerve sheath lesion (neurilemoma or neurofibroma). Such tumours are rare in relation to the central nervous system where they occur more frequently on spinal than cranial nerves. Origin from a large peripheral nerve is far more common.

Many malignant nerve sheath lesions occur in the context of Von Recklinghausen's neurofibromatosis and have the histological features of a fibrosarcoma (Fig. 5.18). S-100 staining may be positive in a proportion of cells of some tumours (Fig. 5.19) but negativity in many reduces its value in proving histogenesis. Malignant neurilemomas are difficult to diagnose with confidence since the diagnosis of a neurilemoma depends largely on recognition of tissue patterns which are usually lost in the face of malignancy. Distinction from a malignant fibrous histiocytoma, which may also be composed largely of spindle shaped cells, may be especially difficult, and evidence of origin from a nerve may be of greater value in establishing a diagnosis than the histological pattern.

One distinctive variant is the epithelioid neurilemoma (Figs. 5.20–5.22) which consists of cords and sheets of cells, with an epithelial appearance, in a collagenous matrix and which usually follows an aggressive course. The cytological resemblances to epithelial cells may make diagnosis difficult but the reticulin pattern (Fig. 5.22) is that of a neurilemoma not a carcinoma (which it may resemble).

The pigmented nerve sheath tumour (Fig. 5.23) combines features of a nerve sheath tumour with the presence of melanin. It may resemble a malignant melanoma, and distinction may depend on demonstrating origin from a nerve. Not all examples are malignant and the presence of melanin in a nerve sheath tumour does not equate with malignancy which is diagnosed on the basis of high cellularity, atypia and mitotic activity. It is difficult to generalise regarding behaviour but local recurrence seems to be a greater risk than metastasis.

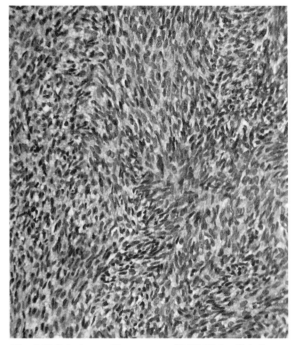

Fig. 5.18 Spinal neurofibrosarcoma. (F 22) High cellularity and mitoses identify this fibrosarcoma which arose in a pre-existing neurofibroma. PS HE × 205

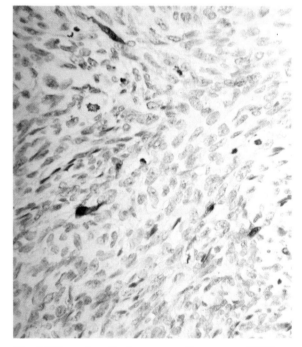

Fig. 5.19 Lateral popliteal nerve neurofibrosarcoma. (F 32) Only a small proportion of tumour cells contain S-100 protein. PS IP S-100 × 320

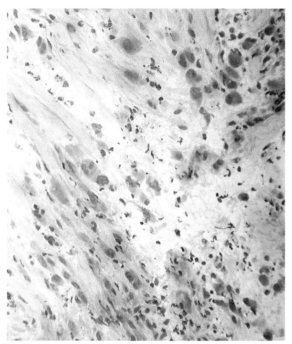

Fig. 5.20 Fifth nerve epithelioid neurilemoma. (M 50) Large tumour cells resembling those of a carcinoma are infiltrating collagen bundles. CS HE × 205

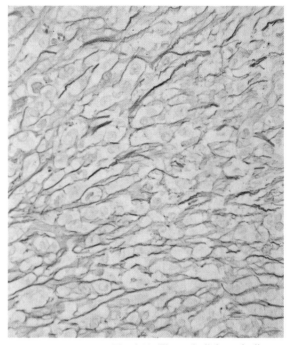

Fig. 5.22 Same case as Fig. 5.20. The pericellular reticulin pattern is characteristic and a useful distinguishing feature from carcinoma. PS RETIC × 320

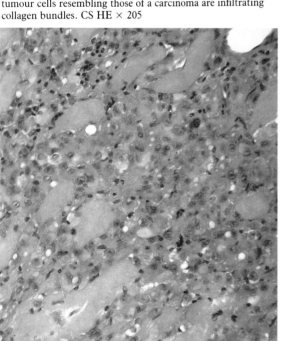

Fig. 5.21 Same case as Fig. 5.20. Distinction from an amelanotic melanoma or carcinoma may be difficult if areas of typical neurilemoma are not present. PS HE × 205

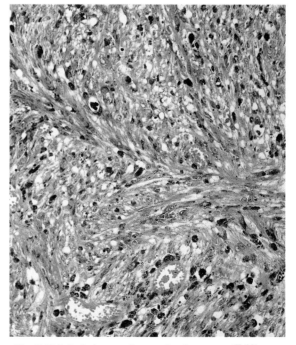

Fig. 5.23 Spinal pigmented nerve sheath tumour. (F 32) Origin from a nerve and the absence of malignant features distinguish this from a melanoma. PS HE × 128

FURTHER READING

Blatt J, Jaffe R, Deutsch M, Adkins J 1986 Neurofibromatosis and childhood tumors. Cancer 57:1225–1229

Bojsen-Moller M, Myhre-Jensen O 1984 A consecutive series of 30 malignant schwannomas. Survival in relation to clinico-pathological parameters and treatment. Acta Pathologica Microbiologica et Immunologica Scandinavica Sect A 92:147–155

Editorial 1987 Neurofibromatosis. Lancet i:663–664

Erlandson RA 1985 Melanotic schwannoma of spinal nerve origin. Ultrastructural Pathology 9:123–129

Franks AJ 1985 Epithelioid neurilemoma of the trigeminal nerve: an immunohistochemical and ultrastructural study. Histopathology 9:1339–1350

Graham DI, Paterson A, McQueen A, Milne JA, Urich H 1975 Melanotic tumours (Blue naevi) of spinal nerve roots. Journal of Pathology 118:83–89

Herrera GA, de Moraes HP 1984 Neurogenic sarcomas in patients with neurofibromatosis (von Recklinghausen's disease). Virchows Archiv (Pathol Anat) 403:361–376

Leslie MD, Cheung KYP 1987 Malignant transformation of neurofibromas at multiple sites in a case of neurofibromatosis. Postgraduate Medical Journal 63:131–133

Matsonou H, Shimoda T, Kakimoto S, Yamashita H, Ishikawa E, Mukai M 1985 Histopathologic and immunohistochemical studies of malignant tumors of peripheral nerve sheath. Cancer 56:2269–2279

Sayed AK, Bernhardt B, Perez-Atayade AR, Bannerman RM 1987 Malignant schwannoma in siblings with neurofibromatosis. Cancer 59:829–835.

Weiss SW, Langloss JM, Enzinger FM 1983 Value of S-100 protein in the diagnosis of soft tissue tumors with particular reference to benign and malignant Schwann cell tumors. Laboratory Investigation 49:299–308

NOTES

6 LYMPHORETICULAR TUMOURS

Lymphomas presenting as tumours of the central nervous system are encountered in two major forms. Firstly as an intrinsic primary lesion, usually within the cerebral hemisphere, and secondly as secondary involvement by an extrinsic deposit that may be the first indication of more widespread disease. In this latter circumstance the site most commonly involved is the spine, although cerebral and cerebellar metastatic deposits, lesions confined to the meninges and subgaleal masses are all encountered. All types of lymphoma may involve the central nervous system although non-Hodgkin's lymphomas of B-cell type predominate in both intrinsic and extrinsic tumours. Metastatic spread to the central nervous system or its coverings in the later stages of an already diagnosed lymphoma is not unusual but meningeal involvement (either as a discrete mass or a diffuse infiltrate) is far commoner than the formation of intrinsic tumour deposits. T-cell tumours are less common but those that present with spinal cord compression are less likely to be part of a disseminated lesion and therefore have a better prognosis.

The classification of lymphomas has undergone many changes over the past 15 years and is subject to continuing revision. The Kiel classification of non-Hodgkin's lymphomas is probably the most widely used with a fundamental division into high and low grade tumours and further subdivisions depending on the nature of the neoplastic cells. Reference to local practice with regard to further subdivision or classification is advised so that management can be standardised and communication with oncologists aided.

Intrinsic cerebral lymphoma is an uncommon tumour previously categorised as a microglioma, but now recognised as being of lymphoreticular origin and sharing the features of extracerebral lymphomas. A range of variants may therefore occur conforming to the diagnostic categories of the latter but certain features, relating largely to their pattern of infiltration, are common to all. Distinction between subtypes of non-Hodgkin's lymphomas is rarely possible, or indeed necessary, intraoperatively the final classification should depend on full examination of all available material.

Lymphomas are composed of non-cohesive cells which, in smears (Fig. 6.1) or touch preparations, separate to show recognisable lymphoid characteristics of size, nuclear morphology and nucleo-cytoplasmic ratio. High grade lesions will often also show considerable pleomorphism and frequent mitoses. In these tumours individual cell death (apoptosis) may be marked although confluent zonal necrosis is less common than in anaplastic carcinomas which may resemble lymphomas cytologically (Fig. 14.7). One characteristic that distinguishes lymphomas from most other tumours is the widespread infiltration by tumour cells of vessel walls which may be visible in cryostat sections (Fig. 6.2). This results in a characteristic expansion of perivascular spaces by tumour cells (Fig. 6.3) which infiltrate and separate the reticulin of both the adventitia and media of the vessel wall. The neuropil may also be diffusely infiltrated by malignant cells (Fig. 6.4), and a considerable astroglial response may result.

Although lymphomas usually produce mass lesions they may be extremely poorly demarcated due to widespread infiltration by tumour cells. As a result surgical specimens may derive from the junctional zone between tumour and normal brain. Small peripheral biopsies from the edge of a tumour may be difficult to interpret, and distinction from an inflammatory lesion may be especially problematic. In the latter the mixed nature of the cells should be a guide, but final distinction may rest on the demonstration that the cells are, or are not, monoclonal by appropriate immunohistochemical methods. Where the diagnosis of lymphoma is made intraoperatively the retention of unfixed tissue in liquid nitrogen is recommended so that subsequent investigation of phenotype for the purpose of classification (by analysis of surface antigens that do not survive routine processing) can, if necessary, be performed.

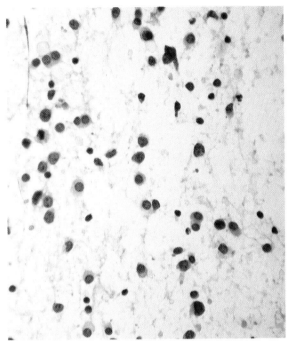

Fig. 6.1 Malignant lymphoma, centroblastic. (F 55) Pleomorphic neoplastic lymphoid cells are well separated and show no tendency to cluster. SP HE × 400

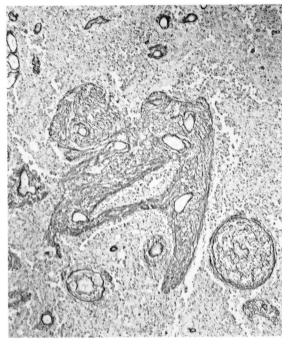

Fig. 6.3 Malignant lymphoma, immunoblastic. (M 26) Blood vessels infiltrated by tumour show expansion of their perivascular connective tissue sheath. PS RETIC × 80

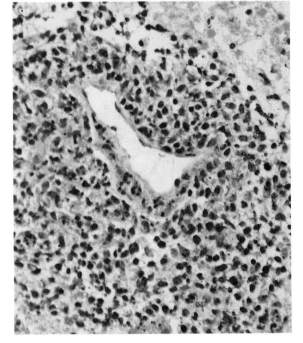

Fig. 6.2 Malignant lymphoma, centroblastic. (M 67) Infiltration of this vessel wall by tumour cells is a hallmark of cerebral lymphoma. CS HE × 320

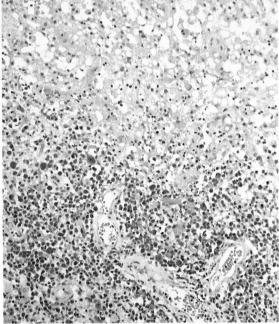

Fig. 6.4 Malignant lymphoma, centroblastic. (M 55) Brain (top) adjacent to infiltrating tumour shows oedema and astrocytic prominence. PS HE × 128

Extrinsic lymphomas usually present as a direct consequence of secondary involvement of the central nervous system or its coverings, particularly (but not exclusively) in relation to the spinal cord. Any form of Hodgkin's or non-Hodgkin's lymphoma may be encountered (Figs. 6.5–6.8). The pattern of the tumour may be distorted by an imposed architecture resulting from infiltration of connective tissue, but the malignant cells can be readily separated by smearing or by use of touch preparations.

A lymphoma can be distinguished from metastatic carcinoma by the failure of cells to form structured aggregates in smears and the absence of specific epithelial features on frozen sections (gland formation, mucin or keratin production).

Biopsies from spinal locations may be small and tough and so are particularly liable to traumatic artefact. As a consequence a clear distinction between a metastatic small cell carcinoma and lymphoma may be difficult or impossible intraoperatively. In appropriate age groups the differential diagnosis may also include neuroblastoma and extra-skeletal Ewing's sarcoma, but it is unlikely that a confident diagnosis could be made on smears and cryostat sections alone. The diagnosis of both these lesions will be greatly aided by electron microscopy and histochemistry (neurosecretory granules and 'neurone-specific' enolase positivity in the former, and glycogen in the latter) emphasising the need to retain appropriately fixed specimens.

MYELOMA

Solitary myeloma may present as a spinal or paraspinal mass (plasmacytoma), or as a bone defect (cranial or vertebral) sometimes with an associated soft tissue component.

Multiple and solitary lesions consist of a monotypic population of plasma cells whose pleomorphism varies with the degree of tumour differentiation (Fig. 6.9). Myeloma deposits may occasionally contain amyloid or crystals formed from light chain material synthesised by the monoclonal neoplastic plasma cells (Fig. 6.10).

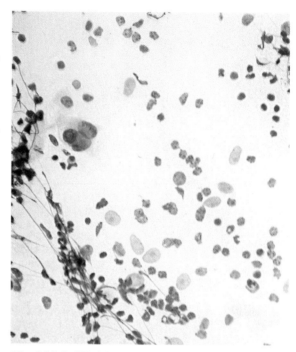

Fig. 6.5 Spinal Hodgkin's disease, mixed cellularity. (M 20) Lymphocytes, multinucleate and atypical cells are some of the components of this tumour. SP HE × 320

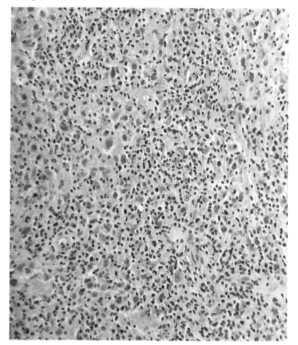

Fig. 6.6 Same case as Fig. 6.5. The predominance of large atypical cells and lymphocytes may make distinction from a non-Hodgkin's lymphoma difficult. CS HE × 205

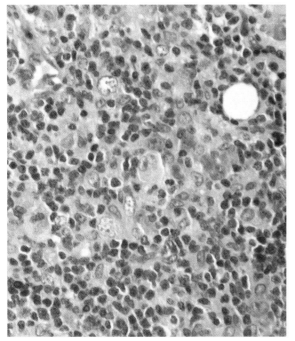

Fig. 6.7 Same case as Fig. 6.5. The finding of binucleate Reed-Sternberg cells (centre) identifies this as Hodgkin's disease. PS HE × 512

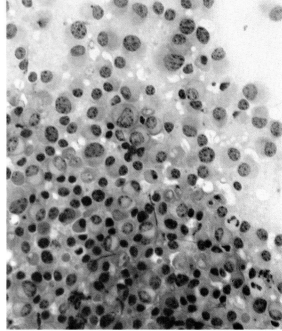

Fig. 6.9 Solitary myeloma of skull. (M 43) The nuclear and cytoplasmic features of these pleomorphic tumour cells are unmistakably plasmacytoid. TP HE × 400

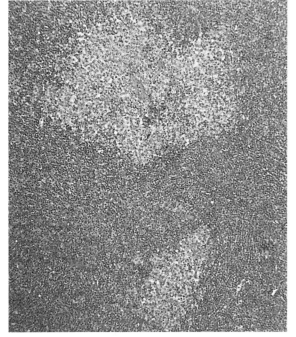

Fig. 6.8 Dural malignant lymphoma CLL type. (F 32) The paler proliferation centres may be confused with the follicles of a follicular lymphoma. PS HE × 80

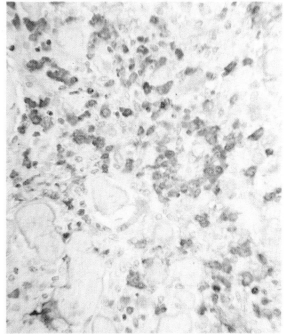

Fig. 6.10 Solitary spinal plasmacytoma. (M 55) Kappa light chains are present in most cells and at the periphery of the spherical deposits of amyloid. PS IP × 320

FURTHER READING

Allengranz AA, Mariani C, Giardini R, Brambilla MC, Boeri R 1984 Primary malignant lymphomas of the central nervous system: a histogenetic and immunohistological study of 12 cases. Histopathology 8:781–792

Bender BL, Mayernik DG 1986 Hodgkin's disease presenting with isolated craniospinal involvement. Cancer 58:1745–1748

Bonnin JM, Garcia JH 1987 Primary malignant non-Hodgkin's lymphoma of the central nervous system. In Pathology Annual Vol. 22 Rosen PR, Fechner RE (Eds) Appleton-Century-Crofts Norwalk Connecticut pp. 353–375

Epelbaum R, Haim N, Ben-Shahar M, Ben-Arie Y, Feinsod M, Cohen Y 1986 Non-Hodgkin's lymphoma presenting with spinal epidural involvement. Cancer 58:2120–2124

Grant JW, Kaech D, Jones DB 1986 Spinal cord compression as the first presentation of lymphoma—a review of 15 cases. Histopathology 10:1191–1202

Hansen OP, Galton DAG 1985 Classification and prognostic variables in myelomatosis. Scandinavian Journal of Haematology 35:10–19

Kalimo H, Lehto M, Nanto-Salonen K, Jalkanen M, Risteli L, Risteli J, Narva EV 1985 Characterization of the perivascular reticulin framework in a case of primary brain lymphoma. Acta Neuropathologica (Berlin) 66:299–305

Kawakami Y, Tabuchi K, Ohnishi R, Asari S, Nishimoto A 1985 Primary central nervous system lymphoma. Journal of Neurosurgery 62:522–527

Knowling MA, Harwood AR, Bersagel DE 1983 Comparison of extramedullary plasmacytomas with solitary and multiple plasma cell tumours of bone. Journal of Clinical Oncology 1:255–262

Kochi N, Budka H, Radaszkiewicz T 1986 Development of stroma in malignant lymphomas of the brain compared with extradural lymphomas. Acta Neuropathologica (Berlin) 71:125–129

Kumanishi T, Washiyama K, Saito T, Nishiyama A, Abe S, Tanaka R 1986 Primary malignant lymphoma of the brain: an immunohistochemical study of eight cases using a panel of monoclonal and heterologous antibodies. Acta Neuropathologica (Berlin) 71:190–196

Lennert K 1981 Histopathology of non-Hodgkin's lymphomas. Springer-Verlag, Berlin.

Levine SB, Bernstein LD 1985 Crystalline inclusions in multiple myeloma. Journal of the American Medical Association 254:1985

Loeffler JS, Ervin TJ, Mauch P, Skarin A, Weinstein HJ, Canellos G, Cassidy JR 1985 Primary lymphomas of the central nervous system: patterns of failure and factors that influence survival. Journal of Clinical Oncology 3:490–494

Murray K, Kum L, Cox J 1986 Primary malignant lymphoma of the central nervous system. Results of treatment of 11 cases and review of the literature. Journal of Neurosurgery 65:600–607

NOTES

7 VASCULAR TUMOURS

The haemangioblastoma can occur anywhere in the neuraxis but is found most commonly in the cerebellar hemispheres and, less frequently, in the spinal cord. Rare supratentorial and multiple lesions have been described but the latter are typically associated with the von Hippel-Lindau syndrome of multiple retinal angiomas, haemangioblastomas, pancreatic cystadenomas and (sometimes) renal carcinoma. Polycythaemia can occur in association with haemangioblastoma, apparently due to secretion of erythropoietin, but there is no histological feature that distinguishes such a tumour from other haemangioblastomas.

Typically the lesion consists of a circumscribed, vascular, cherry-red nodule at the edge of a large cyst, but if lipid-containing cells are abundant the lesion may be tan or yellow. Although frequently associated with a circumscribed cyst spinal lesions may also result in a progressive syringomyelia. The cyst is not an intrinsic part of the tumour but develops as a result of fluid transudation from the component blood vessels into the adjacent neuropil.

The tumour consists of a proliferation of endothelial cells, which form numerous vascular channels of varying size, and a mixed interstitial component of uncertain origin, prominent among which may be lipid-laden cells. Incomplete excision of the lesion will result in persistence of endothelial elements with the capacity for further proliferation and subsequent clinical recurrence. Despite such recurrences true malignant behaviour with metastasis is extremely rare and has to be distinguished from a new, and separate, primary lesion.

While identification of the component vessels is easy when they contain blood they are frequently empty (Fig. 7.1), either as a result of intraoperative ligation of the supplying vessels or compression by stromal cells and so may be difficult to see in a frozen section. The lipid content of the stromal cells may be difficult to appreciate, and some may show eosinophilic staining of their cytoplasm (Fig. 7.2). Coupled with their nuclear pleomorphism (which is of no clinical importance) and cellular anisocytosis, this may lead to the tumour being mistaken for an astrocytoma. A search of other fields should lead to the discovery of tissue that is more obviously formed of capillaries. Even if this is not found, examination of the edge of the tumour at its junction with adjacent brain will show a clear demarcation (Fig. 7.3) which is quite unlike the diffuse infiltration of cerebral tissue by a glial tumour. Identification of the stromal cells as lipid-containing (Fig. 7.4) will also aid diagnosis but if any doubts exist examination of the smear will clearly demonstrate that the lesion is not glial.

Small biopsies from recurrent lesions may be extremely difficult to distinguish from reactive proliferation of small parenchymal and meningeal vessels in the vicinity of a previous operation site, and the presence of lipid-containing macrophages from damaged brain will heighten the resemblance. In reparative states the vessels will all be similar, lacking the variability of size and maturity seen in an haemangioblastoma and, in general, the lipid-laden cells will also be found in relation to adjacent brain rather than restricted to the vascular areas.

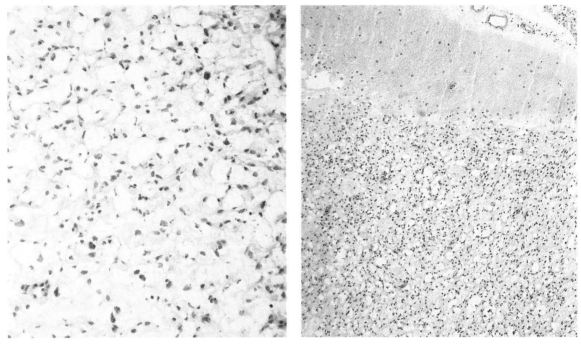

Fig. 7.1 Cerebellar haemangioblastoma. (F 17) Empty capillary channels are inconspicuous although identifiable amongst pale interstitial stromal cells. CS HE × 205

Fig. 7.3 Same case as Fig. 7.1. The clear margin between tumour (below) and cerebellar cortex (above) contrasts with the diffuse edge of an astrocytoma. CS HE × 80

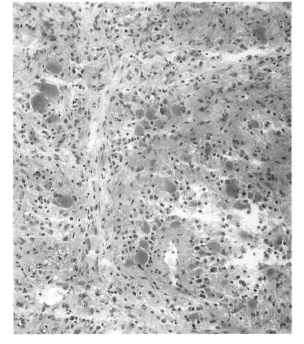

Fig. 7.2 Same case as Fig. 7.1. Elsewhere astrocyte-like stromal cells stain intensely and vascular elements are difficult to identify. CS HE × 205

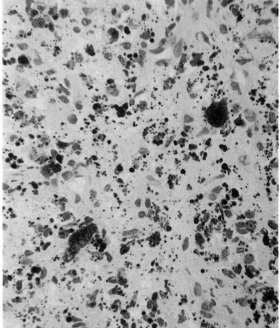

Fig. 7.4 Same case as Fig. 7.1. Neutral lipid is present in many of the stromal cells, but can only be demonstrated on frozen sections. CS ORO × 320

An haemangioblastoma is generally difficult to smear and few cells separate from the tumour tissue. In thin areas of the smear numerous capillaries and capillary buds can be seen with little intervening tissue (Fig. 7.5). Where interstitial cells are prominent they can be identified between vessels and free at the edges of the smear as foamy or eosinophilic lipid-laden cells (Fig. 7.6).

In paraffin sections a range of appearances may be seen with varying proportions of vessels to stroma (Figs. 7.7 & 7.8). The former will vary from thin-walled vascular channels, which in places will amount to sinusoids, to occasional areas of more actively proliferating endothelium where solid endothelial buds will be intermixed with formed capillaries. Although stromal cells may show severe cytological atypia (Fig. 7.9) this has no bearing on tumour behaviour. The interstitium may be formed of loose collagen or filled with the lipid-laden cells described above.

Sometimes the entire lesion may be dominated by stromal cells with the vascular elements reduced to inconspicuous compressed channels (Fig. 7.10). There may be considerable difficulty in distinguishing between such a lesion and a metastasis from a clinically silent clear cell renal carcinoma since stromal cells contain lipid and may also contain glycogen, although the latter is seldom in the quantities found in many renal carcinomas. The arrangement of the 'clear' cells may be a useful feature in that stromal cells in an haemangioblastoma do not form acinar structures (unlike a renal carcinoma), but in a small specimen in which the cells form sheets the problem remains. Immunohistochemical staining for epithelial membrane antigen (EMA) may help to distinguish between the epithelial cells of a clear cell carcinoma (which are usually positive) and the stromal cells of an haemangioblastoma (which do not stain). A proportion of stromal cells in haemangioblastomas stain for GFAP, presumably representing astrocytes secondarily included in an expanding lesion but similar cells can occasionally be found in relation to fibrovascular stroma in metastatic lesions and should be interpreted with caution.

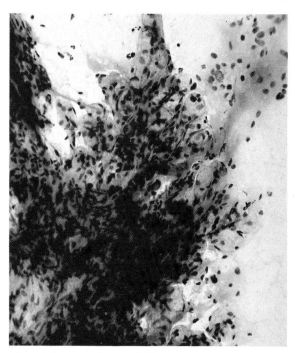

Fig. 7.5 Cerebellar haemangioblastoma. (F 17) Occasionally irregular meshes of capillary loops can be identified at the edge of smears. SP HE × 205

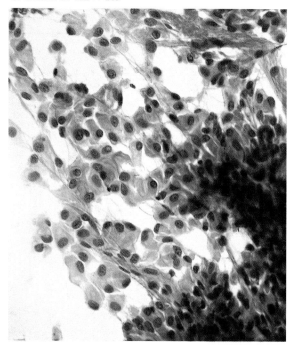

Fig. 7.6 Cerebellar haemangioblastoma. (M 40) If their lipid content is not obvious or not appreciated stromal cells may appear misleadingly epithelial. SP HE × 320

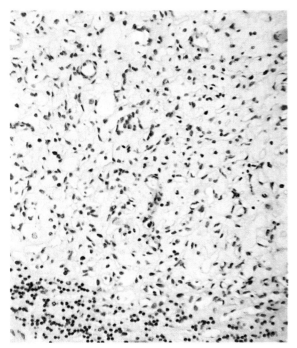

Fig. 7.7 Same case as Figs. 7.1–7.5. Paraffin processing improves the contrast between stromal and vascular elements. CP HE × 205

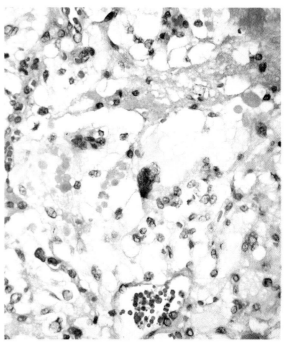

Fig. 7.9 Cerebellar haemangioblastoma. (M 50) Atypical nuclei may be a feature of the stromal element but are of no prognostic significance. PS HE × 320

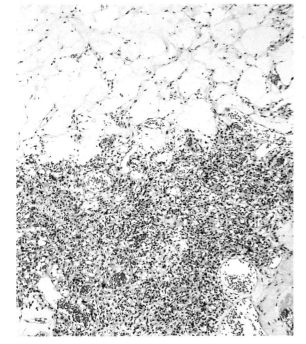

Fig. 7.8 Spinal cord haemangioblastoma. (M 37) Areas with proliferating vessels (below) contrast with zones in which fibrous stroma dominates (top). PS HE × 80

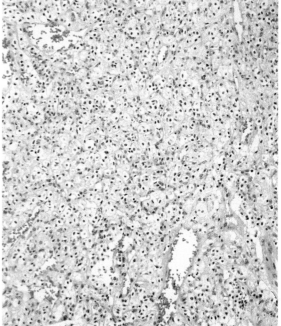

Fig. 7.10 Cerebellar haemangioblastoma. (F 35) Sheets of stromal cells containing lipid, and the vascular pattern, may mimic a renal carcinoma. PS HE × 128

FURTHER READING

Andrew S, Gradwell E 1986 Immunoperoxidase labelled antibody staining in differential diagnosis of central nervous system haemangioblastomas and central nervous system metastases of renal carcinomas. Journal of Clinical Pathology 39:917–919

Deck JHN, Rubinstein LJ 1981 Glial fibrillary acidic protein in stromal cells of some capillary hemangioblastomas: significance and possible implications of an immunoperoxidase study. Acta Neuropathologica (Berlin) 54:173–181

Epstein JI, White CL, Mendelsohn G 1984 Factor VIII-related antigen and glial fibrillary acidic protein immunoreactivity in the differential diagnosis of central nervous system hemangioblastomas. American Journal of Clinical Pathology 81:285–292

Fox JL, Bashir R, Jinkins JR, Al-Mefty O 1985 Syrinx of the conus medullaris and filum terminale in association with multiple hemangioblastomas. Surgical Neurology 24:265–271

Holt SC, Bruner JM, Ordonez NG 1986 Capillary hemangioblastoma: an immunohistochemical study. American Journal of Clinical Pathology 86:423–429

Huson SM, Harper PS, Hourihan MD, Cole G, Weeks RD, Compston DAS 1986 Cerebellar haemangioblastoma and von Hippel-Lindau disease. Brain 109:1297–1310

Mohan J, Brownell B, Oppenheimer DR 1976 Malignant spread of haemangioblastoma: a report on two cases. Journal of Neurology Neurosurgery and Psychiatry 39:515–525

Shimura T, Hirano A, Llena JF 1985 Ultrastructure of cerebellar hemangioblastoma. Some new observations on the stromal cells. Acta Neuropathologica (Berlin) 67:6–12

NOTES

8 PITUITARY TUMOURS

The pituitary adenoma arises from the cells of the adenohypophysis and may present with signs attributable either to hormonal secretion by the component cells or pressure effects on adjacent structures (including the pituitary itself).

A smear from an adenoma (Fig. 8.1) can be distinguished from normal pituitary (Fig. 8.2) by virtue of its monotonous appearance without the regular clustering of cells of differing types that characterises the normal gland. Some cellular pleomorphism (Fig. 8.1) may be a feature although this is not invariable, and cytoplasmic eosinophilia or granules may be visible (Fig. 8.3). The latter may be seen even in a hormonally inactive tumour so it is sufficient to diagnose an adenoma and await paraffin sections to fully characterise it.

Cryostat sections (Figs. 8.4 & 8.5) will reveal either a diffuse pattern with confluent sheets of cells (Fig. 8.4) in a fine enclosing vascular framework, or else a sinusoidal pattern (Fig. 8.5) in which clusters of cells may form small rosettes with central lumina. These two patterns are simply ends of a spectrum and are without obvious clinical significance. An exaggerated sinusoidal pattern may be mistaken for adenocarcinoma if there is a significant degree of cellular pleomorphism, although usually few if any mitoses are seen in an adenoma. Fibrous trabeculae in adenomas are discontinuous in contrast to the connected enclosing pattern of the normal gland.

A tumour with a large suprasellar extension may present as a cerebral mass and be biopsied via a cerebral incision. The sheets of regular cells in a diffuse pattern may be mistaken for an oligodendroglioma (p. 36) although the separation of individual cells that is seen in smears from a pituitary adenoma should alert one to the fact that it is not a glial tumour.

In some lesions calcification may be a feature (Fig. 8.6) and in others (especially, but not exclusively, prolactin secreting) amyloid may form. Neither of these findings appears to have any bearing on behaviour and although the former may give rise to radiological confusion with a craniopharyngioma (p.120) there is unlikely to be any histological difficulty.

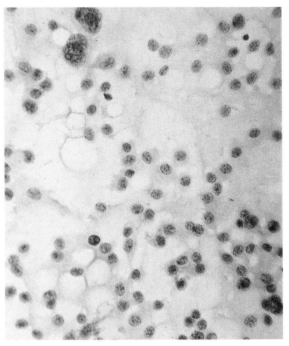

Fig. 8.1 Chromophobe adenoma. (F 60) The majority of cells are palely stained and of the same size although scattered large cells are not unusual. SP HE × 320

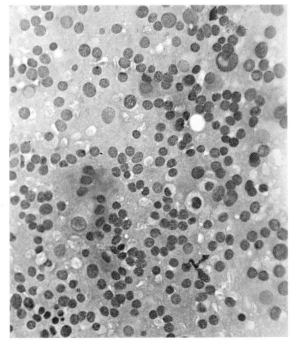

Fig. 8.2 Normal pituitary. (F 36) The mixture of chromophobe, basophil and acidophil cells is reflected in variation in size and staining properties. SP HE × 320

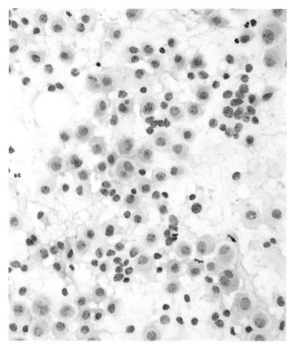

Fig. 8.3 Acidophil adenoma. (F 34) The mixture of larger, clearly acidophilic, and smaller chromophobe cells reflects variable hormonal content. SP HE × 320

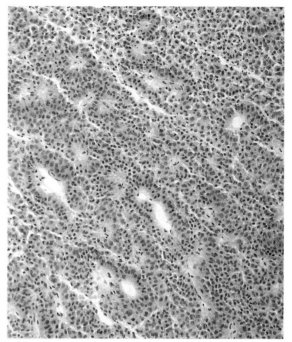

Fig. 8.5 Chromophobe adenoma. (M 76) Sinusoids and rosettes, often alongside blood vessels, are features of a sinusoidal growth pattern. CS HE × 128

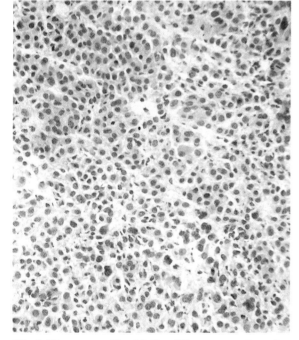

Fig. 8.4 Same case as Fig. 8.1. In a diffuse pattern of growth cells of uniform size are enclosed by a scarcely visible vasculature. CS HE × 205

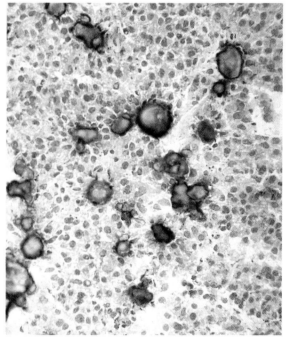

Fig. 8.6 Chromophobe adenoma. (F 36) Although this degree of calcification is unusual smaller numbers of calcospherites are not uncommon. CS HE × 205

The distinctions between the two typical architectural patterns are usually clearer in paraffin sections (Figs. 8.7 & 8.8) but most tumours show a mixture of forms and cellular staining.

By conventional staining techniques tumours are classified as chromophobe, acidophil or basophil. Acidophil tumours stain pink with eosin (Fig. 8.9) and orange with Orange G, basophil lesions stain mauve with haematoxylin and magenta with periodic acid/ Schiff (Fig. 8.10), while chromophobe cells show minimal cytoplasmic staining. Misleading staining may result from artefacts of fixation and handling (intense acidophilia results from surgical compression artefact). Rapidly secreting tumours may retain little, if any, demonstrable hormone so it is not uncommon to find clear clinical evidence of hormone activity with a chromophobe tumour. Conversely, evidence of hormone production (especially prolactin) may be revealed by immunohisto-chemistry without overt clinical signs. Mixed hormone production by tumours is rare with the exception of combined growth hormone and prolactin synthesis (apparently in different cells). Growth hormone secret-ing tumours are usually acidophil (or chromophobe) and ACTH tumours basophil, but immunohistochemistry (Fig. 8.11) and electron microscopy will enable iden-tification of specific hormones.

The cells of an adenoma are naturally infiltrative, and invade residual adenohypophysis and adjacent tis-sues. The histological finding of infiltration by tumour cells is therefore common and its extent may determine the clinical course. In common with many endocrine tumours, cellular pleomorphism (Fig. 8.10) is a feature without clear connotations of malignant behaviour, although it is prudent to draw attention to it, if it is conspicuous, to ensure careful clinical follow-up. The histological diagnosis of carcinoma of the pituitary is based on the presence of mitotic activity (Fig. 8.12) and lesions that metastasise usually show this feature. Distant metastasis is, however, an extremely rare phenomenon and may occur from a tumour which is histologically a typical pituitary adenoma, making con-fident prediction of behaviour difficult.

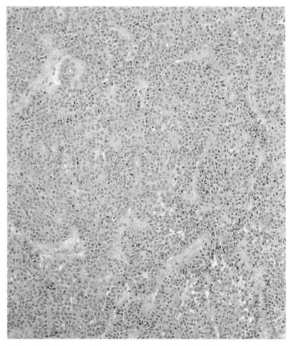

Fig. 8.7 Chromophobe adenoma. (M 49) A diffuse growth pattern shows cell sheets of varying size with a fine intervening vascular stroma. PS HE × 128

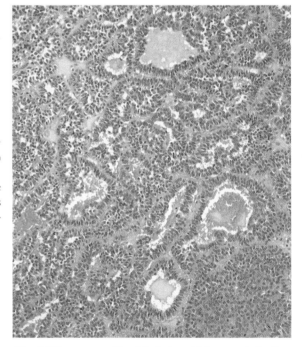

Fig. 8.8 Same case as Fig. 8.7. A sinusoidal pattern is focally prominent but merges with a diffuse area (below). PS HE × 128

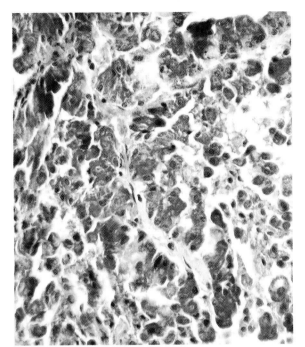

Fig. 8.9 Basophil adenoma in Nelson's syndrome. (F 25) . Tumour cells stain with PAS but immunohistochemistry is necessary to identify hormone product. PS PAS/OG × 320

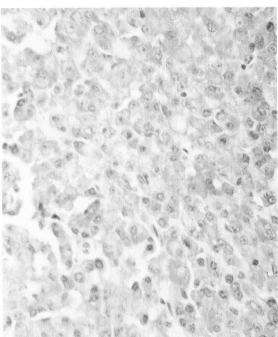

Fig. 8.11 Same case as Fig. 8.10. Specific staining for growth hormone shows considerable intercellular variation in hormone content. PS IP × 230

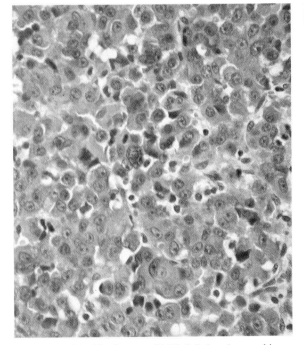

Fig. 8.10 Acidophil adenoma. (F 53) Cellular pleomorphism is often more obvious in acidophil tumours but does not reliably correlate with clinical behaviour. PS HE × 320

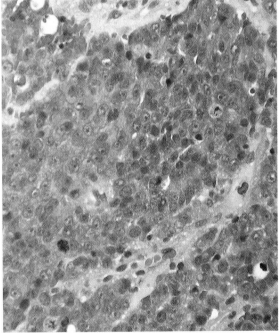

Fig. 8.12 Pituitary carcinoma. (F 58) The high mitotic count indicates malignant change in this recurrent tumour although metastases are not inevitable. PS HE × 320

The term granular cell tumour embraces a heterogeneous group of lesions with a common histological feature, namely the presence of granular cells, which may have a variety of histogenetic origins. They are unusual lesions of uncertain origin although extraneural examples and those attached to cranial nerves are believed to be related to the neurilemoma. They have been described in the cerebrum and more typically (although still rare) in relation to the pituitary. There is evidence to suggest that in the former location they arise from astrocytes and in the latter from cells of the posterior pituitary, although whether from neural or glial elements is unclear. In the pituitary region terms such as granular cell myoblastoma, pituicytoma and choristoma have been applied but in the absence of a clear understanding of their possibly diverse origins the term granular cell tumour is to be preferred. It presents a picture of prominent granular cells with a varying population of spindle cells (Fig. 8.13). Some of the granules stain with PAS and lipid stains suggesting a lipochrome nature, but sometimes melanin (which is also present in the normal posterior pituitary) may be detected.

Other tumours occurring in the pituitary region (craniopharyngiomas, germinomas and sellar cysts) are usually distinctive enough to present few difficulties in differential diagnosis. Problems may be encountered with the distinction between a pituitary adenoma and a carcinoma (Fig. 8.14) which may be infiltrating from a nasal sinus or metastatic from a distant primary. Cytokeratins are present in pituitary adenomas which reduces their value in distinguishing an adenoma from a well differentiated metastatic carcinoma although carcinomas rarely smear with the same uniformity as a primary pituitary tumour. Many carcinomas, however, express epithelial membrane antigen and electron microscopy will usually reveal typical membrane bound granules in pituitary adenomas, even if they are chromophobe in routine preparations.

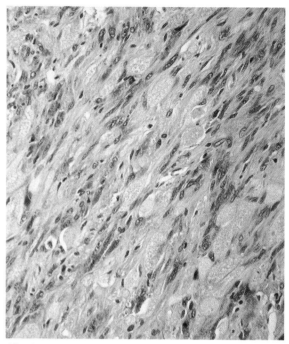

Fig. 8.13 Intrasellar granular cell tumour. (M 58) Prominent granular cells containing lipid and, in some cases, melanin are intermixed with spindle cells. PS HE × 205

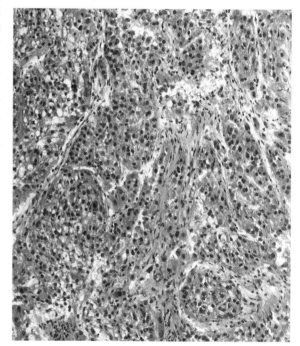

Fig. 8.14 Infiltrating nasopharyngeal adenocarcinoma. (M 59) A trabecular pattern of infiltration may mimic a pituitary adenoma. CS HE × 128

FURTHER READING

Dickson DW, Suzuki KI, Kanner R, Weitz R, Weitz S, Horoupiian DS 1986 Cerebral granular cell tumour: immunohistochemical and electron microscopic study. Journal of Neuropathology and Experimental Neurology 45:303–314

Esiri MM, Adams CBT, Burke C, Underdown R 1983 Pituitary adenomas: immunohistology and ultrastructural analysis of 118 tumours. Acta Neuropathologica (Berlin) 62:1–14

Fan KJ, Pezeshkpour G, Tarfighi J 1985 Pituitary granule cell tumours: an immunohistologic study (Abstract). Journal of Neuropathology and Experimental Neurology 44:309

Horvath E, Kovacs K 1986 Identification and classification of pituitary tumours. In: Cavanagh JB (ed) Recent Advances in Neuropathology 3. Churchill Livingstone, Edinburgh, ch. 4, p. 75–93

Kobrine AI, Ross E 1973 Granular cell myoblastomas of the pituitary region. Surgical Neurology 1:275–279

Kubota T, Kuroda E, Yamashima T, Tachibana O, Kabuto M, Yamamoto S 1986 Amyloid formation in prolactinoma. Archives of Pathology and Laboratory Medicine 110:72–75

Landolt AM, Kleihues P, Heitz PU 1987 Amyloid deposits in pituitary adenomas. Differentiation of two types. Archives of Pathology and Laboratory Medicine 111:453–458

Laws ER, Scheithauer BW, Carpenter S, Randall RV, Abboud CF 1985 The pathogenesis of acromegaly. Clinical and immunocytochemical analysis in 75 patients. Journal of Neurosurgery 63:35–38

Lloyd RV, Chandler WF, McKeever PE, Schteingart DE 1986 The spectrum of ACTH-producing pituitary lesions. American Journal of Surgical Pathology 10:618–626

McKeever PE, Laverson S, Oldfield EH, Smith BH, Gadille D, Chandler WF 1985 Stromal and nuclear markers for rapid identification of pituitary adenomas at biopsy. Archives of Pathology and Laboratory Medicine 109:509–514

Scheithauer BW, Kovacs KT, Laws ER, Randall RV 1986 Pathology of invasive pituitary tumours with special reference to functional classification. Journal of Neurosurgery 65:733–744

Selman WR, Laws ER, Scheithauer BW, Carpenter SM 1986 The occurrence of dural invasion in pituitary adenomas. Journal of Neurosurgery 64:402–407

Symon L, Ganz JC, Burston J 1971 Granular cell myoblastoma of the neurohypophysis. Report of two cases. Journal of Neurosurgery 35:82–89

NOTES

9 PINEAL TUMOURS

Although a variety of tumours may occur in the pineal region, including germinomas (the commonest), teratomas, meningiomas and gliomas, only two tumours, the pineocytoma and the pineoblastoma, are considered to arise from the pineal parenchyma (true pinealomas). There is considerable uncertainty about their histogenesis and while they do appear to be clear clinicopathological entities intermediate forms amay occur.

The pineocytoma usually affects adults in the second half of life and tends to grow by local expansion without metastasis although meningeal dissemination is described in children. The component cells may form rosettes around a central zone of fibrillar eosinophilic matrix, a structural differentiation that may resemble the lobular architecture of the normal pineal gland (Fig. 9.1) although it may not be apparent in sections from small biopsies. The cells are small and regular (Fig. 9.2) (although scattered large cells may be seen) and there may be evidence of cellular differentiation to astrocytes or neurones (Fig. 9.3), the latter being associated with a more favourable prognosis.

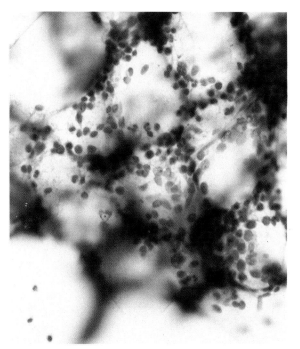

Fig. 9.2 Same case as Fig. 9.1. The cells of the lesion are small and regular and disposed around poorly stained acellular zones. SP HE × 320

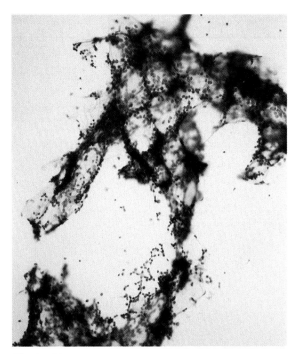

Fig. 9.1 Pineocytoma. (M 18) At low magnification the lobular architecture can be discerned in thick areas of the smear. SP HE × 128

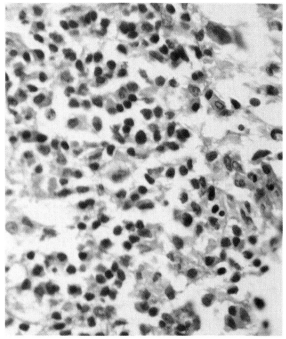

Fig. 9.3 Same case as Fig. 9.1. The large cell at the top of the picture may indicate neuronal differentiation in a relatively uniform cell population. CP HE × 512

This rare tumour is a PNET arising in the pineal and occurs in a younger age group than pineocytomas. Its appearances closely resemble those of PNETs occurring at other sites and it behaves as a more aggressive lesion than the pineocytoma with spread and metastasis through the subarachnoid space. Distinguishing between a pineoblastoma and a metastasis from a cerebellar PNET (medulloblastoma) may be impossible unless there is certainty that the tumour is restricted to the pineal or its environs.

The appearances in smears (Fig. 9.4) are similar to other PNETs (Ch. 4) although pleomorphism is usually greater than in cerebellar lesions and giant cells may occur. The cells are however generally smaller than those of a germinoma (p. 116) which is commoner in this location, and there is no admixture with lymphocytes. Sections (Figs. 9.5 & 9.6) show sheets of primitive cells, occasionally with rosettes of the type seen in cerebellar PNETs (Fig. 4.1). Retinoblastic tubule formation and ultrastructural evidence of retinal differentiation have also been described.

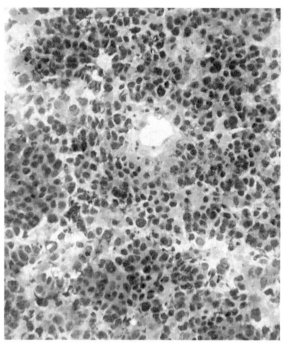

Fig. 9.5 Same case as Fig. 9.4. Pleomorphism is apparent, as is some rudimentary rosette formation, but distinction from other PNETs is difficult. CS HE.× 256

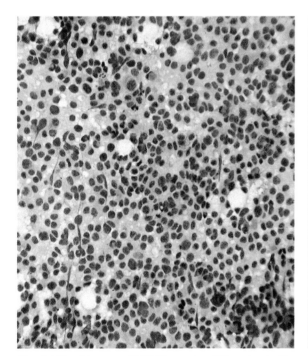

Fig. 9.4 Pineoblastoma. (F 17) Sheets of undifferentiated cells contain scattered giant cells that would be unusual in a cerebellar PNET. SP HE × 205

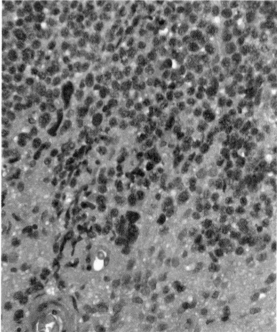

Fig. 9.6 Same case as Fig. 9.4. At the tumour edge where residual pineal (below) is invaded giant cells can be seen. PS HE × 320

FURTHER READING

Borit A, Blackwood W, Mair WGP 1980 The separation of pineocytoma from pineoblastoma. Cancer 45:1408–1418

D'Andrea AD, Packer RJ, Rorke LB, Bilaniuk LT, Sutton LN, Bruce DA, Schut L 1987 Pineocytomas of childhood: a reappraisal of natural history and response to therapy. Cancer 59:1353–1357

Herrick MK, Rubinstein LJ 1979 The cytological differentiating potential of pineal parenchymal neoplasms (true pinealomas). A clinicopathological study of 28 tumours. Brain 102:289–320

Stefanko SZ, Manschot WA 1979 Pinealoblastoma with retinoblastomatous differentiation. Brain 102:321–332

Trojanowsky JQ, Tascos NA, Rorke LB 1982 Malignant pineocytoma with prominent papillary features. Cancer 50:1789–1793

NOTES

10 GERM CELL TUMOURS

Although usually considered as a lesion of the pineal (in which it is the commonest tumour) the germinoma more frequently occurs in a suprasellar location, presumably arising from ectopic germ cells. The appearances are the same as those of gonadal germinomas with a population of large, obviously malignant, tumour cells and an infiltrate of lymphocytes (Figs. 10.1–10.3). The morphology of the malignant component may raise the possibilities of lymphoma, metastasis or (in view of its commoner suprasellar location) pituitary carcinoma. The dual population of cells, the non-cohesive nature, large size and relative uniformity of the neoplastic cells and awareness of its existence, should lead to the correct diagnosis of germinoma. Distinction from a metastatic deposit of a gonadal germinoma cannot be made on histological grounds and such a lesion arising in a site other than the pineal or suprasellar region should be viewed with suspicion.

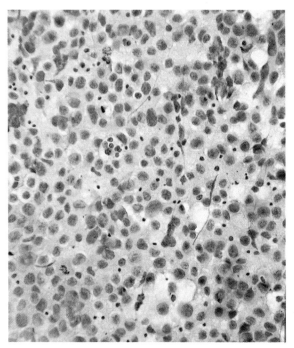

Fig. 10.2 Same case as Fig. 10.1. Lymphocytes are more freely mixed with tumour cells whose prominent nucleoli are better seen in this smear. SP HE × 205

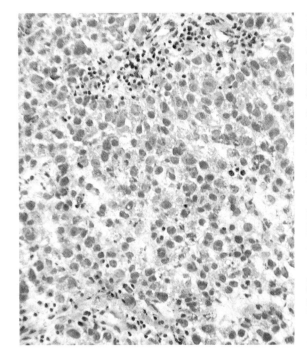

Fig. 10.1 Suprasellar germinoma. (M 22) Sheets of large tumour cells contrast with smaller lymphocytes which are clustered around blood vessels CS HE × 205

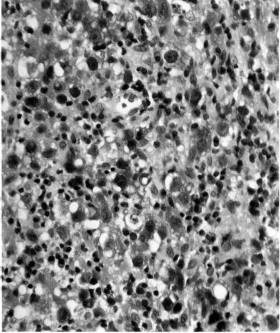

Fig. 10.3 Suprasellar germinoma. (M 17) The neoplastic cells show some pleomorphism and in this case plasma cells are present in the associated infiltrate. PS HE × 320

Teratomas in the central nervous system are rare but most commonly occur in the pineal or suprasellar region in children. Other sites are the spinal meninges (where they are usually benign), the cerebral hemispheres and the posterior fossa (Fig. 10.4). Secondary involvement of the spinal nerve roots may be encountered from primary sacrococcygeal or pelvic lesions. It has been argued that craniopharyngiomas (p. 120) are teratomas but the restriction of their differentiation to stomodaeal epithelium makes this unlikely. Pineal teratomas may be benign or malignant, and tumours with yolk-sac and trophoblastic differentiation occur. Some spinal lesions showing solely endodermal differentiation have been termed 'enterogenous cysts' but usually other lining cells are seen (Fig. 10.5). Malignant cerebral teratomas (Fig. 10.6) contain elements from all germ layers although neuroectoderm may be especially prominent. This may lead to a misdiagnosis of medulloepithelioma (p. 75) but closer examination will usually reveal that other differentiation is present.

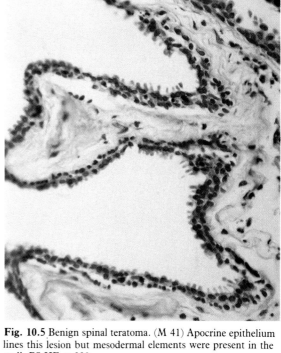

Fig. 10.5 Benign spinal teratoma. (M 41) Apocrine epithelium lines this lesion but mesodermal elements were present in the wall. PS HE × 320

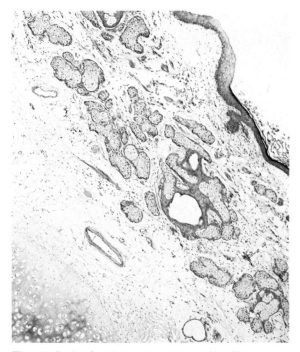

Fig. 10.4 Benign fourth ventricle teratoma. (M 9) The presence of cartilage beneath fully developed epidermis distinguishes this from a dermoid cyst. PS HE × 50

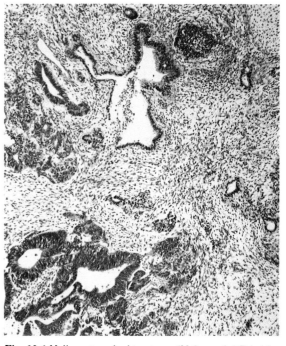

Fig. 10.6 Malignant cerebral teratoma. (M 3 months) Primitive cartilage, mesenchyme, neuroectoderm and endoderm can be identified in this tumour. PS HE × 80

FURTHER READING

Graziano SL, Paolozzi FP, Rudolph AR, Stewart WA, Elbadawi A, Comis RL 1987 Mixed germ cell tumour of the pineal region. Case report. Journal of Neurosurgery 66:300–304

Jennings MT, Gelman R, Hochberg F 1985 Intracranial germ-cell tumors: natural history and pathogenesis. Journal of Neurosurgery 63:155–167

Nakasu S, Handa J, Hazama F, Hirakawa K 1983 Suprasellar yolk-sac tumour in two sisters. Surgical Neurology 20:147–151

Page R, Doshi B, Sharr MM 1986 Primary intracranial choriocarcinoma. Journal of Neurology Neurosurgery and Psychiatry 49:93–95

Shokry A, Janzer RC, Von Hochstetter AR, Yasargil MG, Hedinger C 1985 Primary intracranial germ-cell tumours. A clinicopathological study of 14 cases. Journal of Neurosurgery 62:826–830

NOTES

11 EPITHELIAL TUMOURS AND MAL-DEVELOPMENTAL TUMOUR-LIKE LESIONS

This tumour is of uncertain derivation but has been interpreted as arising from stomodaeal epithelial inclusions. The finding of areas resembling odontogenic epithelium (or lesions of it) or buccal mucosa, and the rare presence of entire teeth, support this view. It typically presents as a suprasellar or infundibular mass, frequently calcified and often cystic.

The characteristic appearance is 'adamantinomatous' (Fig. 11.1–11.3) where a defined basal layer merges with a loose network of cells forming a characteristic pattern. Keratinous whorls (or 'pearls') may form (Fig. 11.2) in which calcium may deposit and other areas, especially if cystic, may be more obviously squamous (Fig. 11.4). The tumours grow by expansion and insinuation into the adjacent brain and often form a cyst that fills the third ventricle and obstructs the aqueduct. The surrounding gliosis is not infrequently coupled with fibrosis which results in an exceedingly tough outer zone from which surgical biopsies may derive. Trapped fragments of neoplastic epithelium may be poorly preserved or disrupted by an inflammatory response that will further confuse the histological appearances (Fig. 11.5). Where there is no inflammatory component the dense gliotic tissue with Rosenthal fibres may closely resemble a low grade pilocytic astrocytoma (p. 14) and careful examination is required if diagnostic epithelial elements are not to be missed.

Cystic areas of the tumour are usually lined by squamous epithelium (Fig. 11.4) and although this may show minimal surface keratinisation, histological and conceptual distinction from a sellar or epidermoid cyst may be difficult. Where the initial management consists of cyst aspiration a thick fluid resembling engine oil is often obtained. The appearances result from the breakdown of red blood cells, tumour cells and brain tissue to give a fluid rich in cholesterol crystals which can be seen in wet smears viewed under polarised light (Fig. 11.6). Caution should be exercised in making a firm diagnosis on this basis alone; the appearances are consistent, or compatible, with a craniopharyngioma, but may be seen in other cystic sellar and suprasellar lesions.

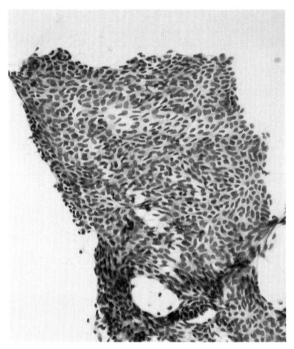

Fig. 11.1 Craniopharyngioma. (M 15) The epithelial nature of the tissue is well seen in smears although architectural detail is lacking. SP HE × 205

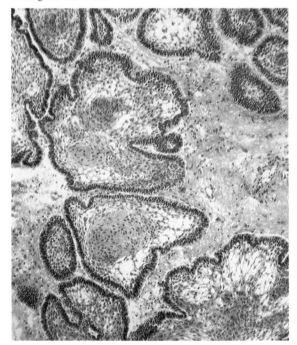

Fig. 11.2 Craniopharyngioma. (M 52) The well-defined basal layer, adamantinomatous pattern and keratin pearls are obvious in this section. CS HE × 80

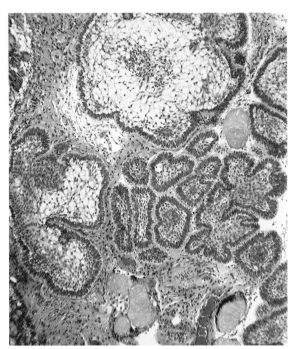

Fig. 11.3 Same case as Fig. 11.2. At the edge of the tumour isolated keratinous masses (below) have provoked gliosis and a giant cell response. PS HE × 80

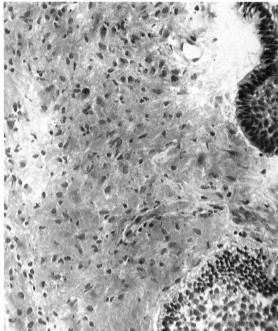

Fig. 11.5 Same case as Fig. 11.2. Tissue from the vicinity of the tumour may show a mixture of reactive astrocytes, Rosenthal fibres and inflammatory cells. CS HE × 205

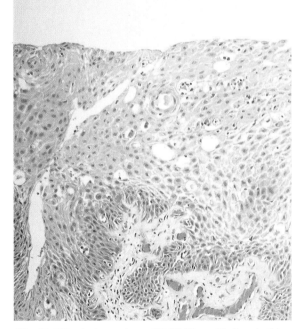

Fig. 11.4 Craniopharyngioma. (M 53) The epithelium in this cyst wall is squamous but there is keratinisation only of single cells and not the surface (top). PS HE × 128

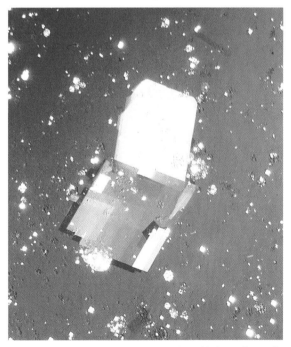

Fig. 11.6 Cystic craniopharyngioma. (F 2) Cholesterol crystals are easy to recognise under polarised light but are not diagnostic. Wet smear × 205

This is an ill-defined group of lesions which may be intra- or suprasellar in location and may be related to the craniopharyngioma. They are lined by a predominantly squamous epithelium (Fig. 11.7) which may also contain ciliated, columnar or even mucous cells (Fig. 11.8). These are termed Rathke's pouch cysts and, while many are asymptomatic, they may rupture or haemorrhage evoking a proliferative fibrous reaction, often with many foreign body giant cells (Fig. 11.9) and cholesterol crystals. These lesions are rarely diagnosed preoperatively being confused with craniopharyngioma or pituitary adenoma. The presence of ciliated cells on a smear is not diagnostic since these may derive from nasal sinuses (breached by the transphenoidal approach or by a primary neoplasm) and clear information as to the source of the biopsy must be obtained. Often the lining epithelium is totally destroyed and the presence of a cyst can only be inferred by the response to its contents.

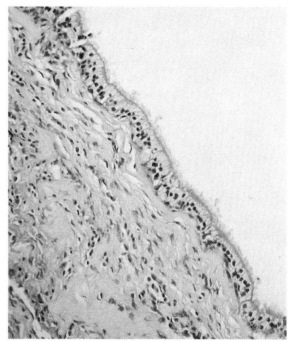

Fig. 11.8 Intrasellar cyst. (F 18) Well developed respiratory epithelium with ciliated and mucous cells covers a dense outer fibrous wall. PS HE × 205

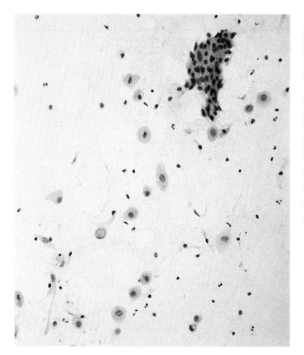

Fig. 11.7 Suprasellar cyst. (F 2) The epithelial lining cells show non-keratinising squamous maturation. SP HE × 205

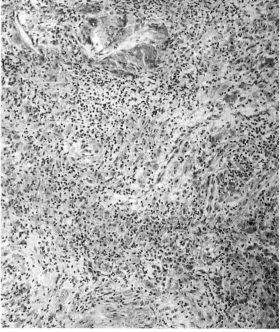

Fig. 11.9 Same case as Fig. 11.8. An area where the lesion has been disrupted shows a vigorous foreign-body giant cell reaction to released cyst contents. CS HE × 128

The colloid cyst is typically located in the third ventricle attached to the ependymal roof or the base of the choroid plexus. It may simply be an inclusion cyst formed by herniation of choroidal or ependymal epithelium into the adjacent connective tissue although similarities with the lining epithelium of Rathke's cysts has lead to the suggestion that it develops from displaced endoderm.

In structure this is a simple cyst with an inner epithelial layer, a fibrous outer wall and mucinous contents (colloid). The lining is usually a single layer of cells which may be ciliated, simple cuboidal or mucus secreting (Figs. 11.10 & 11.11). Cells will be apparent in smears (Fig. 11.12), and a cryostat section may demonstrate the fibrous outer layer of the cyst wall although surgical artefact or poor specimen orientation may result in few cells being visible. Few lesions are likely to be mistaken for a colloid cyst, although clinically the differential diagnosis may include intraventricular meningioma, choroid plexus papilloma or metastasis.

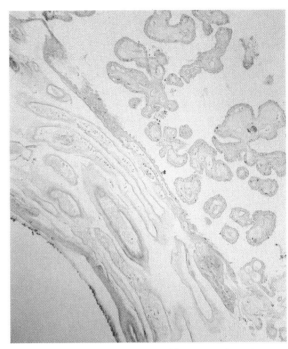

Fig. 11.11 Same case as Fig. 11.10. Mucus secreting cells lining the cyst (below left) contrast with the non-staining cells of the choroid plexus (above). PS AB/PAS ×80

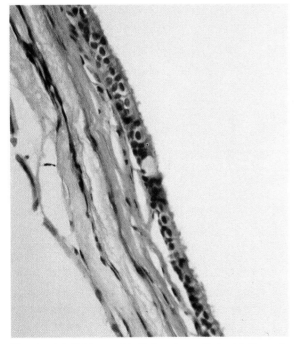

Fig. 11.10 Colloid cyst. (M 67) Pseudostratified epithelium of cuboidal, mucus secreting and ciliated cells lies on a thin fibrous wall. PS HE × 320

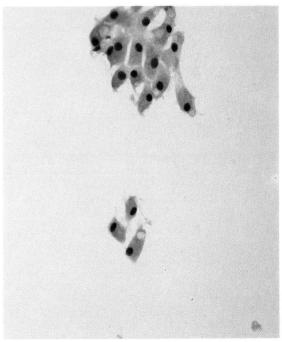

Fig. 11.12 Colloid cyst. (M 55) In a smear cells of differing types may be found, but no architecture is ever discernible. SP HE × 320

Dermoid cysts are characterised by a lining epithelium (which is usually stratified, squamous and keratinising) from which develop epidermal appendages in the form of sweat glands, sebaceous glands or hair follicles. Whilst some of these may represent benign teratomatous lesions the majority are probably developmental inclusions. They tend to be midline in location, to occur with greater frequency in children and there is a frequent association with dermal and osseous defects, especially in the spinal cord where they are commoner than epidermoid cysts. In contrast to the latter they are enclosed in a relatively thick fibrous capsule and so are far more clearly defined. Although often within the subarachnoid space they may be extradural or even intraosseous.

Histologically the lining epithelium consists of the mature keratinising squamous epithelium of normal epidermis with appendage development (Fig. 11.13), but without the mesodermal and other elements of a benign teratoma.

Epidermoid cysts are lined by keratinising squamous epithelium without dermal appendage development. They are found in older patients than dermoid cysts and are usually situated laterally within the cranial cavity, most commonly in relation to the cerebello-pontine angle or the floor of the middle or anterior fossae.

Because it is usually less well encapsulated than a dermoid cyst an epidermoid cyst may extend quite widely within the subarachoid space insinuating itself between existing structures making removal difficult. In consequence the pathologist may be asked to examine material that consists solely of cyst contents, rather than cyst wall, precluding a definitive diagnosis. The latter depends on the presence of a typical lining epithelium (Fig. 11.14), but smears are likely to show either epithelial cells, without any features of malignancy, or simply keratin squames. In the latter case distinction from the contents of a dermoid cyst or even a cystic craniopharyngioma cannot be made.

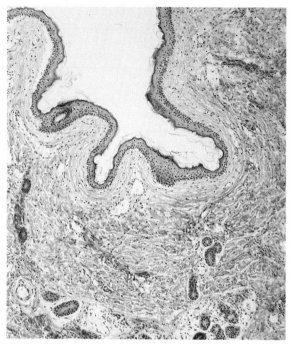

Fig. 11.13 Dermoid cyst from region of anterior fontanelle. (M 4 months) Mature keratinising squamous epithelium forms dermal appendages in this lesion. PS HE × 80

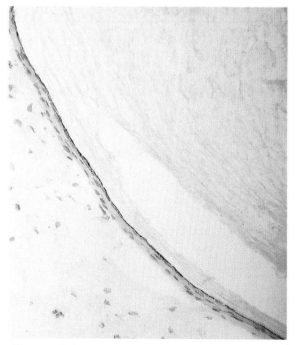

Fig. 11.14 Infundibular epidermoid cyst. (M 27) A thin layer of squamous epithelium with a prominent granular layer abuts on gliotic brain (left). CS HE × 205

FURTHER READING

Berger MS, Wilson CB 1985 Epidermoid cysts of the posterior fossa. Journal of Neurosurgery 62:214–219

Bernstein ML, Buchino JJ 1983 The histologic similarity between craniopharyngioma and odontogenic lesions: a reappraisal. Oral Surgery Oral Medicine and Oral Pathology 56:502–511

Baskin DS, Wilson CB 1984 Transphenoidal treatment of non-neoplastic intrasellar cysts. A report of 38 cases. Journal of Neurosurgery 60:8–13

Friede RL, Yasargil MG 1977 Supratentorial intracerebral epithelial (ependymal) cysts: review, case reports and fine structure. Journal of Neurology Neurosurgery and Psychiatry 40:127–137

Lizczak T, Richardson EP, Philips JP, Jacobson S, Kornblith PL 1978 Morphological, biochemical, ultrastructural, tissue culture and clinical observations of typical and aggressive craniopharyngiomas. Acta Neuropathologica (Berlin) 43:191–203

Petito CK, DeGirolami U, Earle KM 1976 Craniopharyngiomas. A clinical and pathological review Cancer 37:1944–1952

Ryder JW, Kleinschmidt-DeMasters BK, Keller TS 1986 Sudden deterioration and death in patients with benign tumours of the third ventricle area. Journal of Neurosurgery 64:216–223

Shuangshoti S, Roberts MP, Nesky MG 1965 Neuroepithelial (colloid) cysts. Pathogenesis and relation to choroid plexus and ependyma. Archives of Pathology and Laboratory Medicine 80:214–224

Steinberg GK, Koenig GH, Golden JB 1982 Symptomatic Rathke's cleft cysts. Journal of Neurosurgery 56:290–295

NOTES

12 PARAGANGLIOMA

Paragangliomas encountered in relation to the central nervous system arise from receptor cells in the wall of the jugular vein (the glomus jugulare near the jugular foramen), from paraganglia related to the ninth (tympanic branch) and tenth (auricular branch) cranial nerves, and in relation to the cauda equina.

Tumour location will largely determine the presenting signs which may be due to pressure on cranial nerves within the petrous temporal bone (which may be extensively eroded), to middle ear involvement, to intracranial extension as a cerebellopontine mass or, in spinal examples, to pressure on nerve roots.

The architecture of the tumour (Fig. 12.1) is reminiscent of the structure of a normal paraganglion with nests of tumour cells within a fine vascular framework. In intracranial lesions there may be considerable distortion due to infiltration of bone and connective tissue and small clusters of cells, or even individual cells, may lie admixed with small vessels within a dense connective tissue matrix (Fig. 12.2). The result may be a resemblance to infiltrating carcinoma and although the cells of a paraganglioma lack features of malignancy (Fig. 12.3) some nuclear atypia may be seen in recurrent lesions that have been treated by radiotherapy. Deeply infiltrating meningiomas may present in relation to the middle ear (Fig. 3.2) and be mistaken clinically for a glomus jugulare paraganglioma, but the presence of whorls in smears and the lack of the fine vascular framework should identify the former. The tendency of cells to form clusters, and their granularity, may cause a resemblance on cryostat sections to a pituitary adenoma, although the cells of the latter are usually smaller in sections and smear more readily. Clear information about the site of the lesion and its extent should clarify the issue. Spinal lesions may resemble ependymomas in cryostat sections although the smears of the two lesions are quite distinct (Fig. 2.88). In paraffin sections the architecture of the tumour is usually clearer (Figs. 12.4 & 12.5) and neurosecretory granules can be demonstrated by silver stains (Fig. 12.6) or 'neurone-specific' enolase activity.

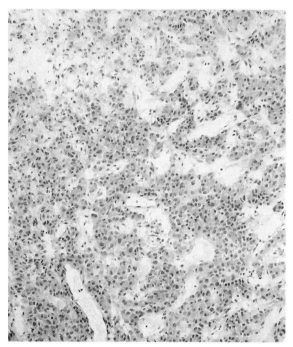

Fig. 12.1 Cauda equina paraganglioma. (M 29) The regular pattern of cells and the relationship to vessels may be mistaken for an ependymoma. CS HE × 128

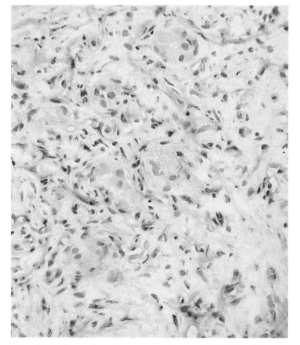

Fig. 12.2 Glomus jugulare paraganglioma. (M 36) Small groups of infiltrating tumour cells are difficult to identify amidst fibrovascular stroma. CS HE × 205

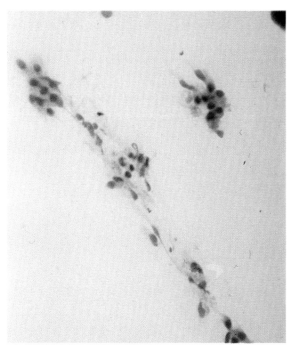

Fig. 12.3 Same case as Fig. 12.2. The few cells that result from smears are regular, cuboidal or columnar, and tend to remain in small groups. SP HE × 320

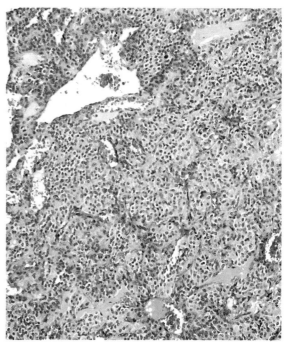

Fig. 12.5 Same case as Fig. 12.1. The 'packeting' of tumour cells by blood vessels is much more obvious than in cryostat sections. PS HE × 128

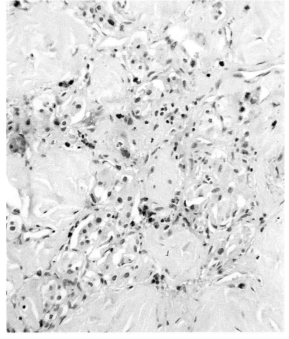

Fig. 12.4 Same case as Fig. 12.2. In paraffin sections the distinction between islands of tumours cells and stroma is clearer. PS HE × 205

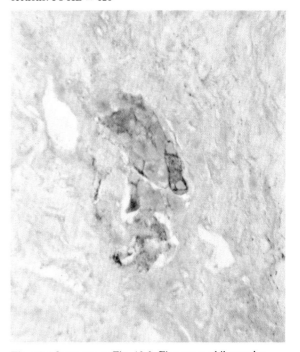

Fig. 12.6 Same case as Fig. 12.2. Fine argyrophil granules identify the tumour cells as being of neuroendocrine nature. PS ChS × 512

FURTHER READING

Anderson JR, Gulan RW 1987 Paraganglioma of the cauda equina: a case report. Journal of Neurology Neurosurgery and Psychiatry 50:100–103

Hatfield PM, James AE, Schulz MD 1972 Tumours of the glomus jugulare. Cancer 30:1164–1168

Ironside JW, Royds JA, Taylor CB, Timperley WR 1985 Paraganglioma of the cauda equina: a histological, ultrastructural and immunocytochemical study of two cases with a review of the literature. Journal of Pathology 145:195–201

Lack EE, Cubilla AL, Woodruff JM 1979 Paragangliomas of the head and neck region. A pathologic study of tumours from 71 cases. Human Pathology 10:191–218

Sonneland PRL, Scheithauer BW, LeChago J, Crawford BG, Onofrio BM 1986 Paraganglioma of the cauda equina region: clinicopathologic study of 31 cases with special reference to immunocytology and ultrastructure. Cancer 58:1720–1735

NOTES

13 CHORDOMA

Although the chordoma is an uncommon primary tumour of bone arising from notochordal remnants, presentation due to secondary involvement of the nervous system occurs so frequently that separate consideration is justified. Approximately two-fifths of all cases arise in the sacrococcygeal region, one-third in the rest of the vertebral column and the remainder in the skull base.

Biopsies present a variety of histological appearances that may in part reflect the effects of sampling rather than biological variants, although chondroid differentiation is associated with a longer natural history.

The tumour may smear poorly but characteristic cells will usually be extracted (Fig. 13.1). While the most striking cell form is the physaliferous (soap bubble) cell, whose bubbly cytoplasm is, in part, due to the presence of mucin (Fig. 13.2), this may not be numerous in its classical form, and the cells may have a more uniformly eosinophilic cytoplasm, especially on cryostat sections (Fig. 13.3). Sections show varying proportions of cells and matrix with patterns that have been interpreted as reflecting the differentiating potential of the notochordal cells from which the tumour arises. Cells may be arranged in cords, trabeculae or lobules (Fig. 13.4), or as separated stellate or spindle cells in palely stained matrix (Fig. 13.5) resembling primitive mesenchyme. A chondroid variant is described although it has been argued on the basis of their antigen expression that such tumours are really low grade chondrosarcomas rather than chordomas.

Chordomas express cytokeratins (Fig. 13.6) and epithelial membrane antigen (EMA), and whilst this is of considerable value in distinguishing them from chondrosarcomas (which do not show such expression) it makes distinction from a clear cell, or other, carcinoma difficult, especially in a small biopsy. Chordoma cells contain glycogen which heightens the resemblance to renal carcinoma, but they also express S-100 protein and vimentin, neither of which are usually found in those carcinomas with which chordomas might be confused.

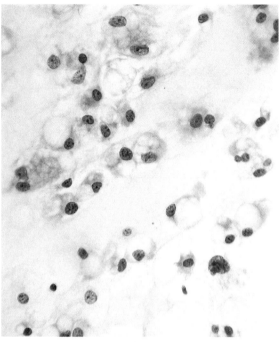

Fig. 13.1 Clivus chordoma. (F 57) When present physaliferous cells are easily recognised in a smear by their cytoplasmic features. SP HE × 320

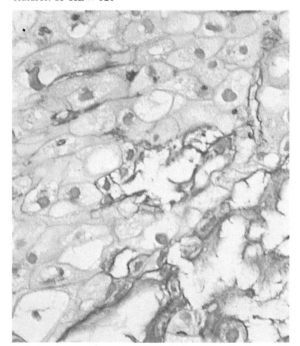

Fig. 13.2 Clivus chordoma. (F 54) Small amounts of mucin can be seen in physaliferous cells, but most is extracellular (bottom). PS AB/PAS/D × 512

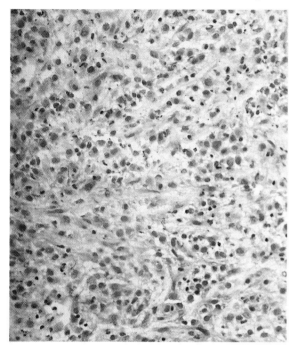

Fig. 13.3 Cervical vertebral chordoma. (M 66) Most cells are eosinophilic and may be difficult to distinguish from those of a primary osteoblastic lesion. CS HE × 205

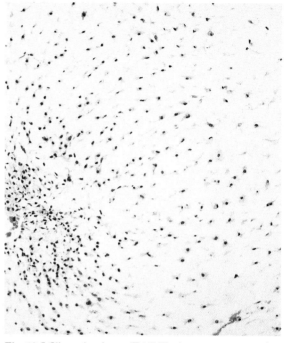

Fig. 13.5 Clivus chordoma. (F 17) The loose arrangement of stellate cells may resemble a chondrosarcoma although pleomorphism is not a feature. PS HE × 128

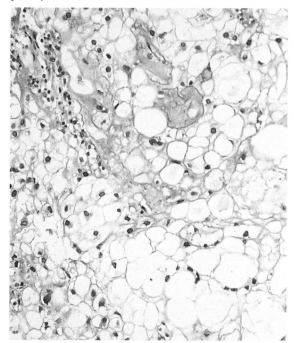

Fig. 13.4 Same case as Fig. 13.2. The dominant cell is physaliferous and forms lobules of tumour in a mucinous matrix. PS HE × 205

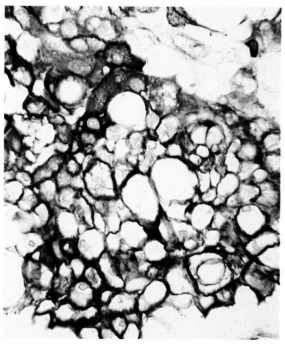

Fig. 13.6 Same case as Fig. 13.2. The expression of cytokeratin distinguishes chordoma from chondrosarcoma but not from carcinoma. PS IP (CAM 5.2) × 320

FURTHER READING

Abenoza P, Sibleyn RK 1986 Chordoma: an immunohistologic study. Human Pathology 17:744–747

Brooks JJ, LiVolsi VA, Trojanowski JQ 1987 Does chondroid chordoma exist? Acta Neuropathologica (Berl) 72:229–235

Coindre J-M, Rivel J, Trojani M, De Mascarel I, De Mascarel A 1986 Immunohistological study of chordomas. Journal of Pathology 150:61–63

Heaton JM, Turner DR 1985 Reflections on notochordal differentiation arising from a study of chordomas. Histopathology 9:543–550

Perzin KH, Pushparaj N 1986 Non-epithelial tumours of the nasal cavity, paranasal sinuses, and nasopharynx: a clinicopathologic study. XIV:Chordomas. Cancer 57:784–796

Rich TA, Schiller A, Suit HD, Mankin HJ 1985 Clinical and pathological review of 48 cases of chordoma. Cancer 56:182–187

NOTES

14 METASTATIC TUMOURS AND SECONDARY INVOLVEMENT

Metastatic tumours of almost any origin may involve the central nervous system but it should be remembered that, even in the face of a clear clinical history of a primary tumour elsewhere, a tumour of the central nervous system may still be a metachronous primary lesion. A significant proportion of metastatic lesions present without clinical evidence of a primary tumour and (rarely) may even occur within a pre-existing cerebral tumour (Fig. 14.1). Presentation may relate to a deposit within the cerebrum or cerebellum, to an extrinsic lesion (frequently dural or extending from bone) compressing the brain or, more frequently, the spinal cord. Involvement by direct extension from an adjacent primary tumour (such as intrinsic bone tumours of the skull or vertebrae, salivary gland tumours and tumours of the nasopharynx) (Fig. 8.14) may also be encountered.

In practice the majority of lesions are epithelial malignancies (including melanomas) whose component cells are joined by desmosomes of varying degrees of development. As a result, whilst single cells separate readily from tumour tissue in smear (or dab) preparations (Fig. 14.2), there is an intrinsic tendency for cells to form cohesive clusters (Fig. 14.3). Sections will reveal any specialized differentiation (Figs. 14.4 & 14.5) (gland formation, keratinisation, mucin, pigment or osteoid production) and intrinsic architectural patterns, but reactive fibrosis or infiltrated connective tissue (especially in the spine) may distort these.

Problems most frequently arise in relation to small biopsies from anaplastic tumours or in the interpretation of reactive glial tissue in the vicinity of a metastatic tumour deposit (Fig. 2.4). There is a very clear demarcation between most metastatic tumours and adjacent brain (Fig. 14.6) with minimal single cell infiltration so that a biopsy may be taken very close to a metastasis without malignant cells being present. Occasionally glioblastomas may show features that are focally indistinguishable from carcinoma (p. 34), but in these circumstances examination of more material, identification of GFAP within tumour cells, or electron microscopy will usually resolve the issue.

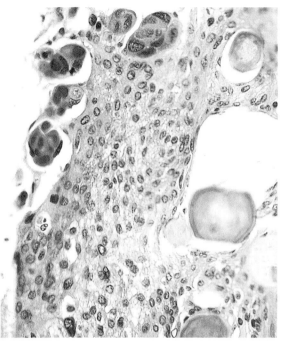

Fig. 14.1 Metastatic breast carcinoma in meningioma. (F 69) Metastatic tumour cells (top left) contrast with smaller more uniform meningioma cells. PS HE × 320

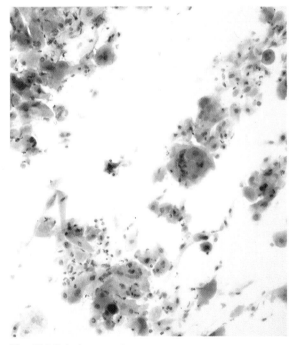

Fig. 14.2 Spinal metastatic squamous carcinoma. (F 69) Clusters of malignant keratinising cells are unmistakably from a carcinoma. SP HE × 128

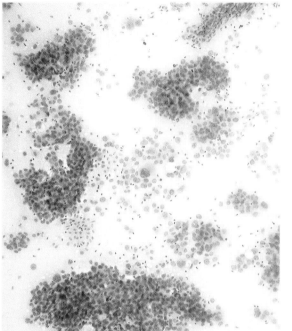

Fig. 14.3 Cerebral metastatic adenocarcinoma. (M 65) Clusters of cells with a background of separated malignant cells are typical of tumours forming acini. SP HE × 80

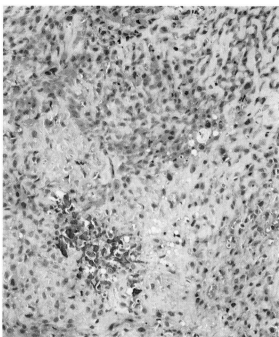

Fig. 14.5 Spinal metastatic osteogenic sarcoma. (F 11) Care must be taken that reactive osteoid related to metastases is not mistaken for tumour. PS HE × 128

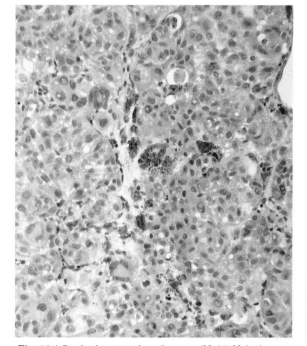

Fig. 14.4 Cerebral metastatic melanoma. (M 64) Melanin pigment was only focally present in this lesion and was barely visible on cryostat sections. PS HE × 205

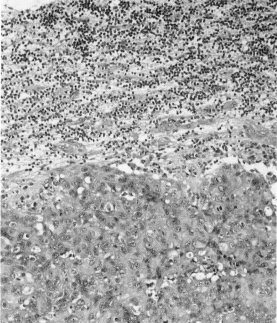

Fig. 14.6 Cerebellar metastatic breast carcinoma. (F 46) The margin between tumour (below) and compressed cerebellar cortex (above) is well defined. PS HE × 128

Intrinsic tumours are more likely to be mistaken for metastasis than the other way round. Small cell glioblastomas (Fig. 2.61) or PNETs (Fig. 4.4) resemble oat cell carcinomas (Fig. 14.7), myxopapillary ependymoma (Fig. 2.100) may mimic adenocarcinoma (Fig. 1.6 & 14.8), haemangioblastomas (Fig. 7.10) may resemble clear cell carcinoma of kidney (Fig. 14.9) if they have a prominent stromal cell component, and choroid plexus carcinoma (Fig. 2.111) may be indistinguishable from a metastatic deposit. Occasionally urothelial tumours show prominent perinuclear haloes and may be confused with an oligodendroglioma. The use of one, or several, of the growing range of available 'markers' of epithelial cells (Fig. 14.10) will usually resolve such problems on paraffin sections. Experience has shown that these are not as specific as was initially hoped and cross-reactions continue to be documented, so wherever possible a 'panel' of markers should be used. A pan-leucocyte marker may be of value when dealing with small cell malignancies although a small proportion of lymphoid tumours fail to stain.

An atypical meningioma (Fig. 3.25–3.27) which has invaded beyond the bone into extracerebral soft tissue may be confused with a carcinoma. Despite the presence of atypical cells and mitoses the general uniformity of the cells seen in a meningioma is quite distinct from the pleomorphism of most carcinomas (Figs. 14.1 & 14.2)

An uncommon form of metastatic involvement of the nervous system seen with leukaemias, lymphomas and carcinomas is a diffuse meningeal infiltration in which malignant cells are usually found in the CSF (Fig. 14.11). Distinguishing cells of a lymphocytic lymphoma or leukaemia from reactive lymphocytes can be difficult if only small numbers are present and full account should be taken of the clinical history. The recognition of carcinoma cells will not usually be difficult but cells from a mucin producing carcinoma may resemble macrophages and be associated with a mixed inflammatory response. In these circumstances staining spare preparations (or restaining the originals) for mucin (Fig. 14.12) will clearly demonstrate the true nature of the cells.

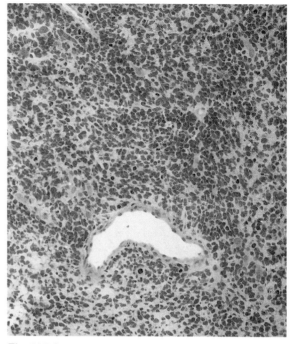

Fig. 14.7 Cerebellar metastatic oat cell carcinoma. (F 66) Cytology and lack of vascular invasion help to distinguish this carcinoma from lymphoma. CS HE × 128

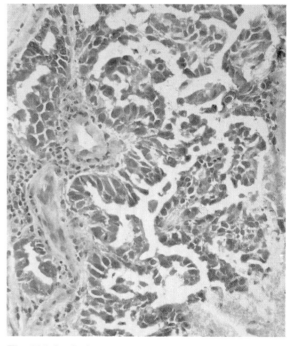

Fig. 14.8 Cerebral metastatic adenocarcinoma. (F 59) Malignant cells form acini and papillae over fibrous stromal cores. CS HE × 205

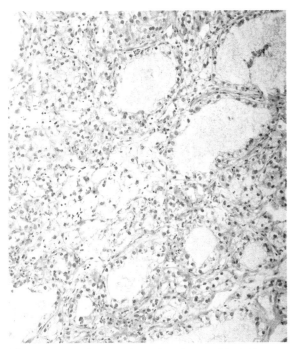

Fig. 14.9 Cerebral metastatic renal carcinoma. (M 66) Tumour cells, which form sheets and line acini enclosed by fine vessels, show minimal pleomorphism. CS HE × 128

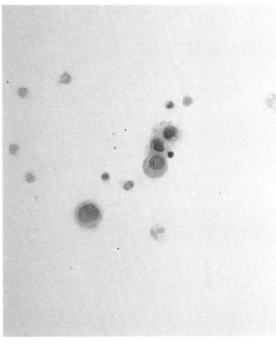

Fig. 14.11 Metastatic breast carcinoma in CSF. (F 35) Large tumour cells with atypical nuclei contrast with reactive lymphocytes and monocytes. CYTO HE × 320

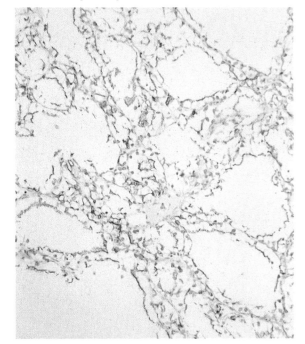

Fig. 14.10 Same case as Fig. 14.9. Epithelial membrane antigen stains tumour cell surfaces and provides an absolute distinction from haemangioblastoma. PS IP × 128

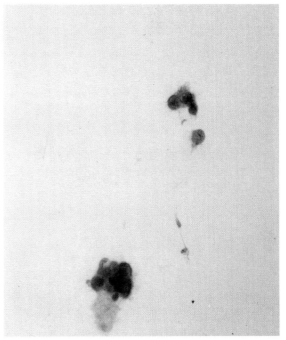

Fig. 14.12 Metastatic gastric carcinoma in CSF. (M 68) Tumour cells resembled macrophages on routine preparations but contain acid mucins. AB CYTO × 320

FURTHER READING

Baumann MA, Holoye PY, Choi H 1984 Adenocarcinoma of prostate presenting as brain metastasis. Cancer 54:1723–1725

Chambers PW, Davis RL, Blanding JD, Buch FS 1980 Metastases to primary intracranial meningiomas and neurilemomas. Archives of Pathology and Laboratory Medicine 104:350–354

Delsol G, Gatter KC, Stein H, Erber WN, Pulford KAF, Zinne K, Mason DY 1984 Human lymphoid cells express epithelial membrane antigen. Implications for diagnosis of human neoplasms. Lancet ii:1124–1129

Galloway PG, Roessman U 1986 Anaplastic astrocytoma mimicking metastatic carcinoma. American Journal of Surgical Pathology 10:728–732

Leong A S-Y 1986 Antibody probes in the diagnosis of anaplastic tumours. I Malignant round cell tumours. Pathology 18:296–305

Murray PK 1985 Functional outcome and survival in spinal cord injury secondary to neoplasia. Cancer 55:197–201

Pamphlett R 1984 Carcinoma metastatic to meningioma. Journal of Neurology Neurosurgery and Psychiatry 47:561–563

Schoenberg BS, Christine B, Whisnant JP 1975 Nervous system neoplasms and primary malignancies of other sites. The unique association between meningiomas and breast cancer. Neurology 25:705–712

Sloane JP, Hughes F, Ormerod MG 1983 An assessment of the value of epithelial membrane antigen and other epithelial markers in solving diagnostic problems in tumour histopathology. Histochemical Journal 15:645–654

Variend S 1985 Small cell tumours of childhood: a review. Journal of Pathology 145:1–26

Yoshimine T, Ushio Y, Hayakawa T, Hasegawa H, Arita N, Yamada K, Jamshidi J, Mogami H 1985 Immunohistochemical study of metastatic brain tumours with astroprotein (GFAP), a glia-specific protein. Tissue architecture and the origin of blood vessels. Journal of Neurosurgery 62:414–418

NOTES

APPENDIX: ANATOMICAL DISTRIBUTION OF TUMOURS

These tables are not intended to be comprehensive but indicate the likelihood of encountering a particular tumour in a particular anatomical region. Tumours in brackets are uncommon or rare.

Table 1 Supratentorial

Adult	Child
Glioblastoma	Astrocytoma
Astrocytoma	(Oligodendroglioma)
Meningioma	(PNET)
Metastasis	(Ependymoma)
(Oligodendroglioma)	(Teratoma)
(Lymphoma)	

Table 2 Infratentorial

Adult	Child
Neurilemoma	Astrocytoma
Meningioma	PNET
Metastasis	Ependymoma
Haemangioblastoma	(Choroid plexus papilloma)
(Ependymoma)	
(Choroid plexus papilloma)	

Table 3 Sellar region and skull base

Pituitary adenoma
Meningioma
Craniopharyngioma
Sellar cyst
(Germinoma)
(Chordoma)
(Paraganglioma)
(Metastasis)

Table 4 Spinal Cord (Intra- and extradural)

Neurilemoma
Meningioma
Metastasis
Myeloma/Lymphoma
Ependymoma
(Astrocytoma)
(Haemangioblastoma)
(Chordoma)

INDEX